Healing Tonics

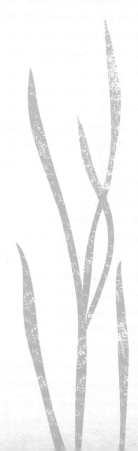

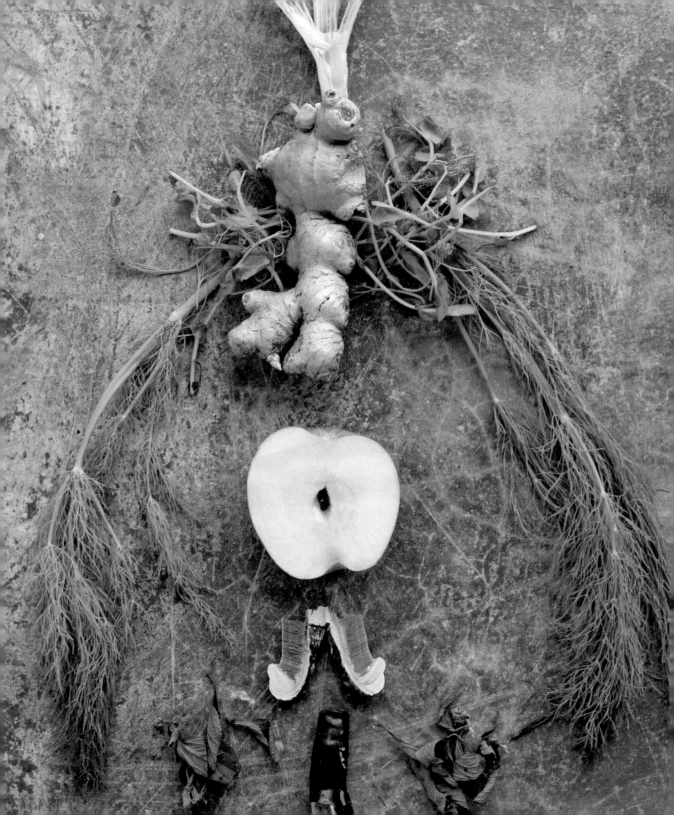

Healing Tonics

Next-Level
Juices, Smoothies, and Elixirs
for Health and Wellness

Adriana Ayales

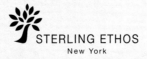

STERLING ETHOS
New York

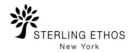

STERLING ETHOS
New York

An Imprint of Sterling Publishing Co., Inc.
1166 Avenue of the Americas
New York, NY 10036

This publication is intended for informational purposes only. This publication includes alternative therapies that have not been
scientifically tested. The publisher does not claim that this publication shall provide or guarantee any benefits, healing, cure,
or any results in any respect. This publication is not intended to provide or replace conventional medical advice, treatment,
or diagnosis or be a substitute to consulting with a physician or other licensed medical or health-care providers. The publisher
shall not be liable or responsible in any respect for any use or application of any content contained in this publication or any
adverse effects, consequence, loss, or damage of any type resulting or arising from, directly or indirectly, the use or application
of any content contained in this publication. Any trademarks are the property of their respective owners, are used for editorial
purposes only, and the publisher makes no claim of ownership and shall acquire no right, title, or interest in such trademarks
by virtue of this publication.

Distributed in Canada by Sterling Publishing
c/o Canadian Manda Group, 664 Annette Street
Toronto, Ontario, Canada M6S 2C8
Distributed in the United Kingdom by GMC Distribution Services
Castle Place, 166 High Street, Lewes, East Sussex, England BN7 1XU
Distributed in Australia by Capricorn Link (Australia) Pty. Ltd.
P.O. Box 704, Windsor, NSW 2756, Australia

For information about custom editions, special sales, and premium and corporate purchases, please
contact Sterling Special Sales at 800-805-5489 or specialsales@sterlingpublishing.com.

Manufactured in Canada

2   4   6   8   10   9   7   5   3   1

www.sterlingpublishing.com

Photography by Jennifer Harter, www.jenniferharterphotography.com
Book Design by Susan Walsh

With all my heart, this book is dedicated to my family.
You have all guided and nourished my heart beyond measure.
To my beloved partner and our baby boy that will continue spreading
the magic of herbs, and to all the aspiring herbalists out there
that are teaching the ancient ways of being in harmony with nature.

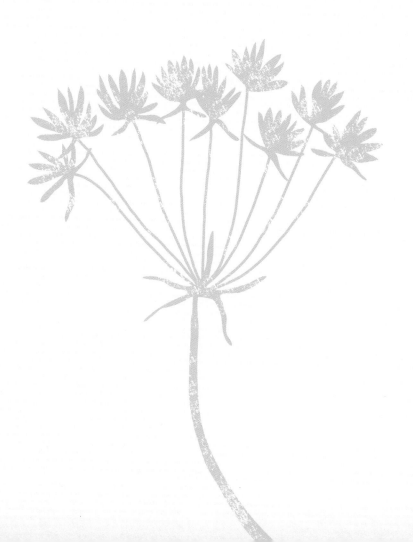

Contents

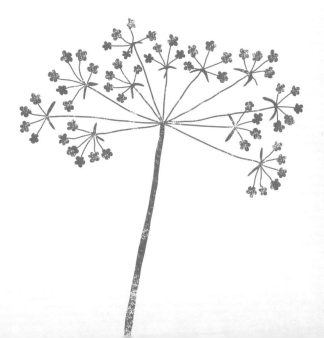

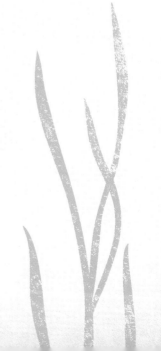

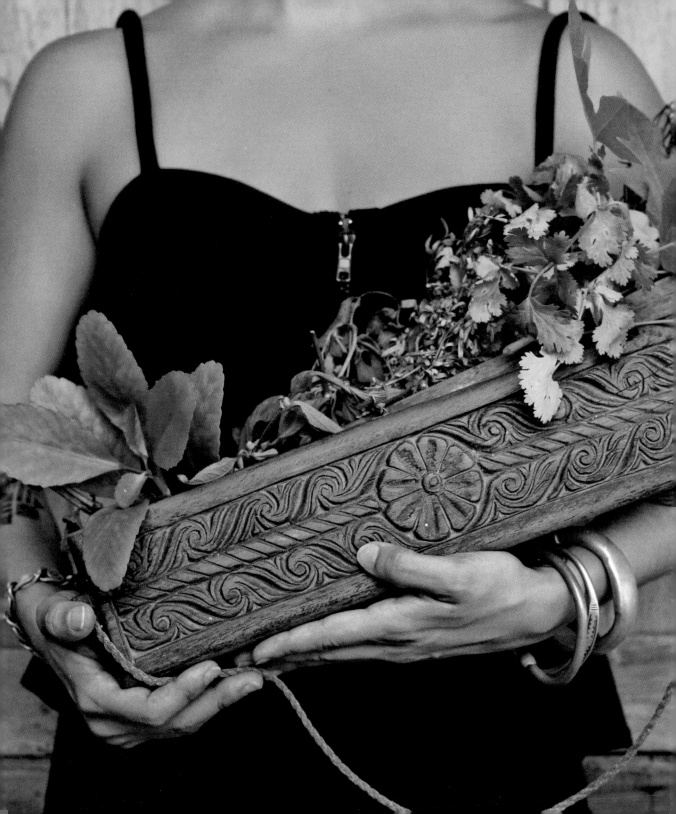

Introduction:
Be Your Own Kitchen Doctor

Creating and living the dream requires so much more than I anticipated. Day by day, holding space, passion, and focus to manifest one's heart's desire is perhaps the most ecstatic and intense journey there is. Doing what we truly love requires a tireless devotion to the mission each of us is here to share. I've learned that when people work from their heart, they are filled with an energy so much bigger than themselves that all there is left to do is follow and listen.

I come from a place where the kitchen pantry is a medicine chest. The superfoods and botanicals found in the rainforest naturally invoke a sensational warmth. The soil itself, rich with out-of-the-ordinary nutrients, evokes soulful sensations. It hosts a huge variety of botanicals, fruits, and foods that can enhance any kitchen with their healthful properties. In the rainforest, even the most common backyard weed is perhaps the next antidote for some serious illness.

I was fortunate to be brought up in the jungle. The auspicious energy of Costa Rica taught me about the magic and miracles of nature. A rainforest kitchen is usually composed of an abundant selection of mouthwatering fruits, extraordinary flowers, colorful spices, and delectable vegetables. It is a wonderland of availability. Born to a line of passionate Costa Ricans, with a strong Lebanese heritage, I was destined to have a kaleidoscopic life. From a young age I was a spiritual seeker constantly driven to find the answers within the mystery of nature. My destined mission as a medicine maker crystallized for me with the powerful teachings my grandmother passed on to me at a young age. My nana was a key figure in my development of intuitive sight; practices applied at a young age taught me to unlock hidden reservoirs within our heritage. We would undertake intuitive practices and psychic meditations that allowed me to see further into the mysticism of healing. I believe that tapping into our body's innate wisdom through practice, grants us the gift of intuitive sight within the inner workings of nature.

As I grew up, I learned from different influential *curanderas* (female folk healers or medicine women) and, yogis. I trained in hands-on healing, herbalism, ethnobotanical traditions, spirit cleansing, and therapeutic cooking. As my practice developed, a voice in me grew louder and louder, and I simply kept following and creating. My focus on vibrant and holistic living through therapeutic herbalism became my total mission.

It is not by accident that we suddenly find ourselves in the places we least imagined, where the inner wilderness happens to flow out of you in a particular time and space. In my case, New York City was indeed that last place I would have imagined I would be living.

Having the high contrast of experiencing both jungles—tropical and urban—nourished me in an unexpected way. As I lived in the city, I would travel to upstate New York to get my dosage of nature while working at a healing kitchen in a retreat center. Meanwhile, I would go back down into the city and continue my private practice as an herbalist in Brooklyn. After seeing many people day after day, sharing common ailments, and needs, I created base formulas that would help the average complaint. These formulas would tackle the common symptomology experienced in today's world: from migranes, to overstressed guts, seasonal allergies, detoxification, insomnia, weight loss, and so on.

Shortly after, I started an herbal company focused on rainforest super tonics and formulas that supported vibrant living. Anima Mundi Herbals became the manifestation of my intention to bring rainforest botanical traditions to the modern world through a product line that transmitted the ancientness and purity of these practices. It was a thrill to see people's responses and healing experiences while taking these formulas. It was mind-blowing to witness miracles and life transformations through adoption of this lifestyle and herbal integration into daily living. About 2 years later, I opened Botica, a modern-day apothecary and cold-press juicery that adopts rainforest herbal formulas into the entire juice, smoothie, and food menu.

My life and work as an herbalist, therapeutic chef, and medicine maker have taught me the importance of preserving and restoring ancient botanical teachings, a crucial part of today's history. My vision is to bring recipes and powerful longevity formulas back into practice by teaching others how to incorporate them into the kitchen. This book protects the seeds of the ancient story through a step-by-step guide on how to alchemize your daily foods with the power of herbal wellness.

In this book you will find traditional recipes that draw upon rainforest traditions, particulary from Costa Rica and the Amazon. As you delve into each recipe, you will discover how to reveal the beauty within yourself through diet, ritual, and lifestyle. You will also find out about the role of vibrant superfoods, tonic superherbs, and the daily psychology of longevity.

These recipes are an expression of rainforest culture, people, and folklore utilizing the curative power of botanicals and superfoods. Most ingredients found throughout these pages reflect what has been revered for decades as basic essentials in daily living. I created these formulas inspired from rainforest magic, to empower your life with vibrant recipes steeped in sacred tradition.

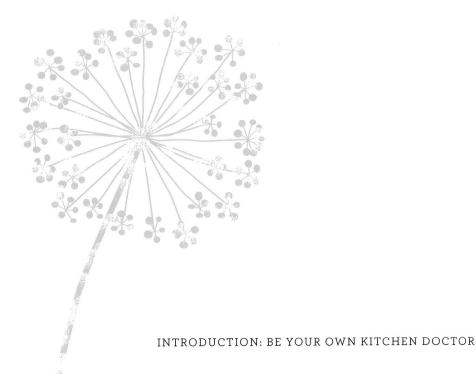

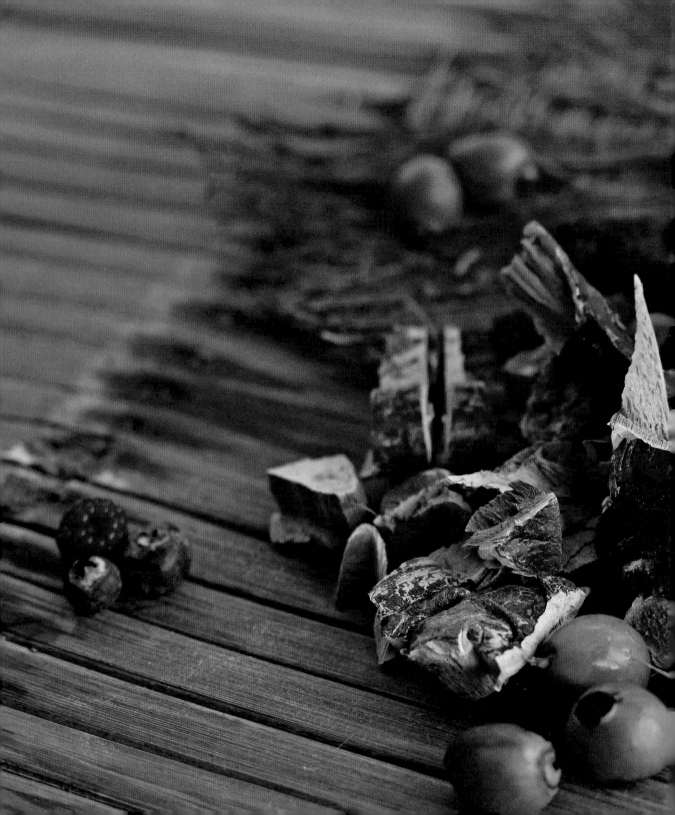

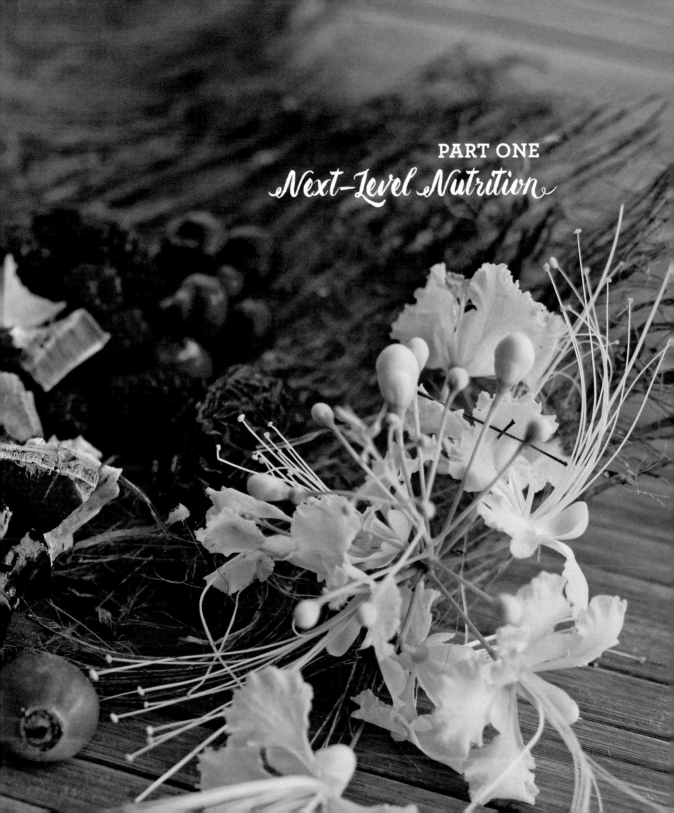

PART ONE

Next-Level Nutrition

THE BASICS

The Power of Medicinal Herbs

It's well known that herbs promote wellness. In fact, the word *drug* originally meant "dried herb." Herbs grow around the world, and their history, is certainly as old as the first plant ever found on Earth. Herbs, in Eastern and Western traditions, have been the central component of traditional healthcare. In the East, as well as in Central and South American native cultures, intricate botanical systems demonstrate the science behind their healing cosmology. Each culture has intensively studied herbs, refining their qualities and abilities through thousands of years of meticulous research.

The earliest written account of humans using medicinal plants dates to around 3000–2000 BCE. Among the most ancient texts are those within Ayurveda in India, as well as Chinese writings depicting the mythology of and psychosomatic response to each plant. Whether by oral or written traditions, each culture is steeped in knowledge of the remarkable power of herbs. Each tradition built a healing cosmology that treats the body as a whole, connecting cosmic to internal aspects as primary sources known to cause change within the body. Such fully developed systems do not need to be refined, but rather translated and adapted into society in more active ways.

The Western mind shifted this integral attention and created a fundamental error—a tendency to treat the disease rather than the patient. If only drugs were made to be prescribed sensitively in accordance to the individual nature of each patient, as in Eastern traditions, then side effects could be avoided.

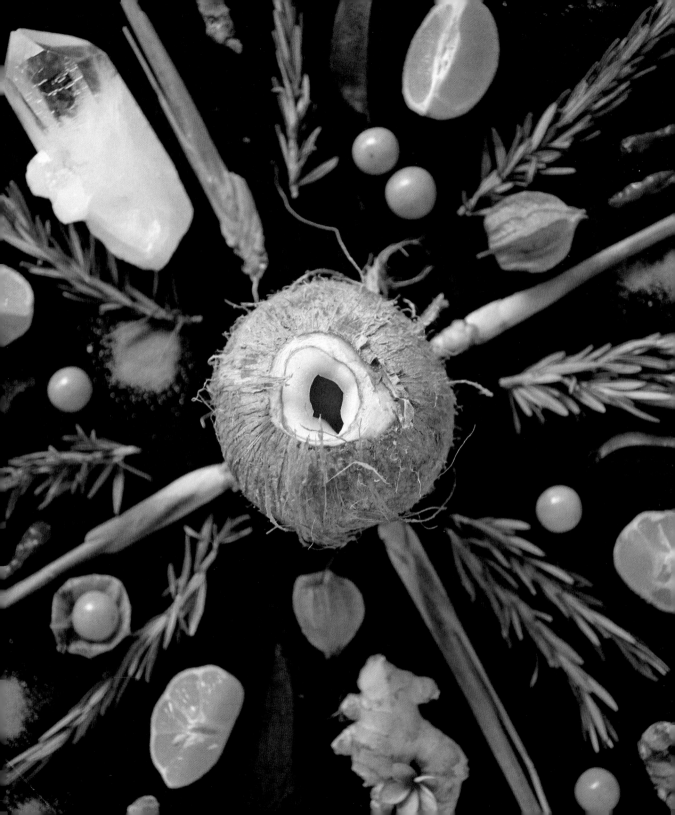

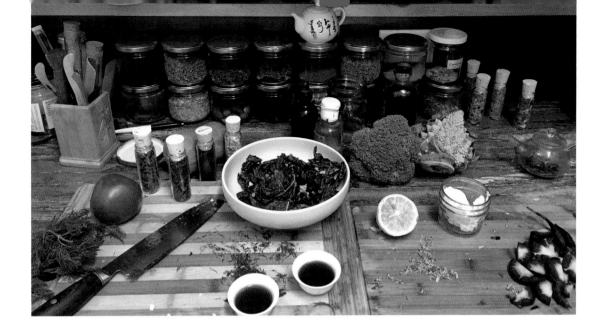

MIND, BODY & HERBS

Some people may have the opinion that the science behind ancient healing techniques is not as refined as today's medicine. In my opinion this makes no sense. If we look at the source of today's medicine, we see that even sophisticated modern medical practices are rooted in prehistoric science—the science of nature. The major difference between the fundamentals of back-in-the-day healing and today's is that our ancestors did not separate the psychospiritual element from the scientific. True pharmacology, as studied by the Mayans, Egyptians, Chinese, and other cultures, integrated the heart and mind into empirical studies. It wasn't a matter of belief; it was simply an undoubted fact in nature that the spiritual and physical bodies were intertwined and both should be addressed. This was essential and not even a question—in fact, if you didn't address this union, it often meant you couldn't compose and formulate for others as a medical practitioner.

Plants exist to transmute light into life. Human beings exist to transmute life into consciousness and love. These three properties—light, life, and love—are one. They are each an expression of the other, three dimensions of the same existence. Plants transmute life into light through photosynthesis. Humans transmute light into consciousness through perception. Through direct perception, the seer is the seen, and the observer is the observed. Bringing this basic understanding as the foundation to your wellness will awaken a higher meaning in your kitchen pharmacy.

e kidneys and ears are shaped simi-
mbryo. The embryo and the later
fetus, grows
in the water
medium,
through
which sound
travels to its
developing areas ears.
In traditional Chinese medicine,
problems of the ears or hearing
may reflect a water element disharmony.
dneys govern the storage of the life
e marrow. People with bone problems
while healthy bones are a healthy
ke, "I feel it in my bones" or "She cries
elationship of the bones to deep emotional
a good time to seek deeper and more
get to those meaningful and emotion-

relates to the sexual organs and the
ly. It rules over the genital and
he urethral and the anal orifices. The
t affects the energy flow during the
the function of the reproductive organs,
ater in the body. Sexual fluids help
sperm and the egg. An excess of sex &
ll as a lack of expression of sexual
kidneys as well as the water balance.
requires giving and receiving, ying + yang,

eridians of the body has the energy
ominantely 2hrs a (for each meridian)
7pm each day.
tion, it has
primarily
gravitational
ly expan-
he moon
tides) and
body +
in, the
principle,
s — the hidden
onal. Like the
roughts and flood

"Within the kidneys, 'essence' is stor
all that is secluded and dormant and
their condition is disclosed in the bone.
—Ch

BLADDER
The bladde
in the pelvis
urine re
The c
to b
if
res
T
em
an
the
at
over
a long
and t
back o
ending a
side of
Tens
easil
area,
well as ne
ing + flexing
clears the ene
a flexible num
In the Ch
are perceive
the life fo
are relate
the cycle
to the Kia
is a chronic

seat of the will", wil
as coming from the Kidn
ambition. Other organs of elimination beside
are lungs, large intestine, and the skin. W
toxins poorly or have too much to handle, the sk
harder to help clear waste; skin rashes are a
Naboru Muramoto feels strongly about kidn
ted from the stress of toxic chemicals and he
This can lead to poor clearly, resulting in ov
(excess fluid volume) placing extra work to the
hemical additives stiffens the vascular sys
high blood pressure and weakening the hear
To evaluate the health of the kidney
color, clarity and tone of skin. Bluish decolo
a water imbalance. The presence of spar
from the vital "life-force" in the kidneys.
examine the texture of u

2

Ancient Juicing Traditions

Until agriculture was developed around 10,000 years ago, all humans got their food by hunting, gathering, and fishing. From laying of the seed to hunting to gathering to preparing, connection to every part of the food cycle was a basic day-to-day reality.

In recorded texts, most of what we find on ancient juicing technology pertains to wine and liquid cleansing and fasting. Many ancient civilizations used liquid dieting and cleansing as a way to enhance their spiritual practice and connection to the gods. Most technology used to create juice actually pressed the fruits, either by hand or with screwing devices that would squeeze the juice out of the fruit. Records suggest that the more pure, unfiltered, and unmodified you can keep the fruit, the more the body and mind will benefit from the therapeutic result.

THE SCREW: THE FIRST PRESS

By the time of ancient Greeks, all simple machines had been invented but one. The last simple machine to be developed was the screw. The screw is based on another simple machine, the inclined plane, yet has the advantage of generating a massive amount of force through circular movement. This simple mechanism has enabled us to lift very heavy loads; to build homes, boats, and modern machines; and, last but not least, to build a juice press!

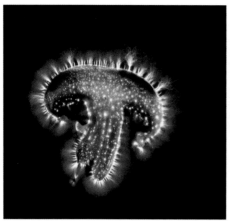

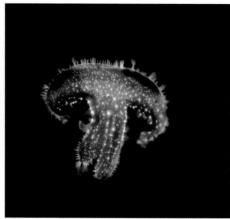

One of the screw's most important uses in ancient times was in the screw press. This device combined two simple machines—the screw and the lever—to magnify force. Ancient people used the screw press primarily to squeeze juice from grapes and oil from olives. (These are two of the greatest things in life!) This particular system did not use heat to extract more oil or juice; it was pure pressure—the result was what we now refer to as "cold-pressed."

THE POWER OF COLD-PRESSED JUICE

The greatness of cold-pressed juice is that it's the most biologically perfect juice. Many believe that adding heat to the process of juicing is what destroys live enzymes and chemical structures that are essential to the human digestive system. The vitality that has been found within a cold-pressed juice is unparalleled. When compared to heat-induced juices, such as those created using centrifugal machines, cold-pressed juice has an overwhelmingly superior nutritional profile.

Any heat over 120°F (48°C) will change the biochemical constituents of any food, primarily because of the enzyme factor. Enzymes are the transformers of the microbiome. They enable constant renewal in the gut and basically help us on a moment-to-moment basis to prevent digestive stagnation. Enzymes are small proteins that contain the intelligence of where to send the nutrients in the body. Without the proper enzyme sources (herbs, raw plant foods), we begin to accumulate undigested materials in our system. This leads to sickness, imbalance, inflammation, digestive distress, and fatigue. Enzymes are available within every cell of the human body—every single part of your body has the potential of being a highly supercharged battery of potential, containing thousands of enzymes! The secret to unlocking some of these dormant enzymes is trace minerals, most found only in essential superfoods and herbs.

Raw cold-pressed juice is a miraculous carrier of medicines. Juice can become the enzymatic medium to gain magnificent mineralization from the medicines added to it. The richer the vehicle to which the medicines are added, the more it will enhance enzyme function, come alive, and masterfully absorb the complexities of the chemistry within the tonics. The more potent the carrier, the deeper the medicine can penetrate tissue and organs. Our ancient ancestors combined medicinal herbs into their food as a staple element in food prep and cooking. These herbs, throughout time, ended up being classified as spices. However, while some herbs contributed to the flavor profiles of the dishes being cooked, there is another set of herbs that are not quite as aromatic as common spices but are essential in enhancing the nutrition of food, and so are classified as spices despite their primary purpose. For example, in Central American cooking, a few leaves of epazote were always added to beans to prevent gas building up in the intestines, help the protein digest more easily, and provide strong antibacterial protection to the body. Although epazote is also known for its pungent, anise-like flavor, it is added primarily for its health properties. A variety of other "spices" have entered our culinary repertoire for similar reasons: adding herbs to your daily food and beverage empowers your body's ability to thrive.

RAW LIVING

During the first ages, humankind subsisted primarily on raw plant foods and raw meats. The prehistoric human diet was mostly leafy foods, nuts, seeds, roots, herbs, and fruits because they were the easiest foods to acquire. People often debate whether humans were originally carnivores, herbivores, or omnivores. The truth is that humans will and can eat almost anything. Our digestive system is able to process almost anything we want. Regardless of our food choices or current dietary plan, food affects the way we think, feel, and behave. When discernment is introduced into one's food choices, a significant physical and spiritual transformation occurs. Real, wholesome, and raw plant-based nutrition has always been around and immediately available within nature. This simple fact signals that the higher the percentage of these wholesome foods we consume, the more vibrant and alive we'll feel.

Your Kitchen as a Sacred Space

If the home were a body, the kitchen would be the reproductive system.
—DEEPAK CHOPRA

The kitchen is a very intimate space. Within it we find the complete set of tools to create the deepest nourishment for the body. The quality of space where we make our nourishment is as vital as the quality of the ingredients used. Beautiful spaces that are sacred to *you*, have the power to create the most healing and nourishing magic possible. The kitchen is like an altar where you cook your prayers and manifestations into what fuels your body. Cleaning and making your meals provides the perfect opportunity to become one with everything on which you focus your awareness. Your kitchen doesn't have to look like all the other kitchens: make it the playground that you've always wanted. Flowers, incense, pictures, crystals, fruits . . . anything! Have it be the place you love to be. I promise you, this will change your life. The simple act of mindfulness to make food and medicine can naturally increase self-love, make a home peaceful, and even lower cortisol levels!

Shifting your awareness to the fact that food is a sacred communion with your self and nature immediately fuels a life of longevity. Think about it: if food is our medicine, then the place of its creation is of utmost importance. In many cultures, the maker of the food is among the most respected people within the community. The person is creating a divine offering for all to enjoy and be in a heavenly place.

Let's start by really looking at your kitchen. What does it need, and how can we optimize it?

COSMIC EVOLUTION
Within the Microcosmic Life of a Plant

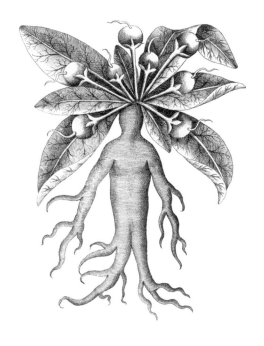

Crown/
Brow
Aether
5

PLANETS=SPIRIT
Main motivating cosmic force.

Heart/
Throat
Air
3

FLOWER=SOUL
Cleanses the psychic environment.

Navel
Fire
1

LEAF=MIND
Draws in the cosmic life force, *qi*.

Sacral
Water
4

SEED-ROOTS=BODY
Integrates the constitutional blue print.

Root
Earth
2

DIAGNOSING YOUR KITCHEN

Cleanliness: Is it cluttered? Is it sterile? Does it have a lot of things? There is a clear connection between a clean kitchen and well-being. Studies have shown that a neat and clean home can actually lower cortisol levels.

Space: Do you have a small or a large kitchen? Is it shared? Do you live alone? Regardless of the space, it is important to have the essentials present in a way that works. If your kitchen is small, keep only what's important in your daily routine out and ready. Everything else that you are not using on a daily basis, or even at all, can be organized or disposed. If your kitchen is big, try not to accumulate too many unnecessary kitchen items; only make space for your favorites and your essentials.

Available Ingredients: How long has each ingredient in your pantry been there? Is the majority of your refrigerator filled with fresh fruit, veggies, or meats? Or is your food mostly canned? Is your kitchen usually full of food, or is it constantly empty? What are the staples in your cupboard and in your refrigerator?

Creative: Are inspirational items on display? Art? Plants? Crystals? Do you host dinner parties? Do you take pleasure in having a guest or two over on a regular basis? Providing a welcoming environment for friends is a great way to maintain the kind of kitchen that we would love for ourselves. By creating a nice atmosphere and great dishes that you know your friends will enjoy, you enliven the space and do your best to impress. Use entertaining as a test to see if you can keep that level of dedication with yourself on a daily basis.

Spiritual Cleansing: How regularly do you energetically clean your home? Do you use sage or other smudges to clear the atmosphere? Keeping a clean and tidy kitchen is great, but sometimes we forget to energetically cleanse it and the rest of the house. This means creating a harmonious *feng shui* environment within your home, as well as keeping a clear atmosphere. Sage, palo santo, juniper, and other sacred smudges clean energy and are actually healthy to keep around. They are strong antibacterial air purifying agents that also are known to clear

bad and stagnant energy. Whether or not you perform spiritual housecleaning in your weekly routine, it's a good idea to give your entire home and body a thorough energetic cleansing.

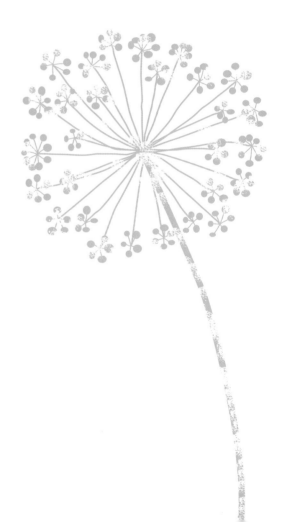

Superfoods and Superherbs: The Food and Medicine of the Future

A new life is dawning in the nutrition world. More and more people are turning to next-level nutrients and foods. There is increasing interest in the benefits of organic foods as well as in natural supplements. We are approaching a critical mass of consumers shifting their purchasing power toward local, pure, and organic products. The formerly cutting-edge world of organics and superfoods is now a mainstream reality shared by people from all walks of life. Now that organic living has become more regular living, people are seeking superfoods and superherbs to add a higher healing element to their diet.

Superfoods are a powerful group of foods that have at least a dozen more unique properties than regular food. They have been seen through the centuries as tonic medicines that can be consumed safely as foods on a daily basis. For example, goji berries have remarkable blood-purifying and mineralizing qualities, great liver-cleansing properties, anti-aging chemistry, and a megaload of antioxidants.

Superherbs, on the other hand, have even more super tonic and adaptogenic properties with extraordinary healing gifts. Superherbs can be added safely to daily living, unlike other botanical powerhouses, yet they tend to be added to diets in lower doses due to their intensive tonic potency. For example, reishi mushroom helps support immune, heart, lung, and kidney function while assisting with rejuvenation in the brain and connective tissue.

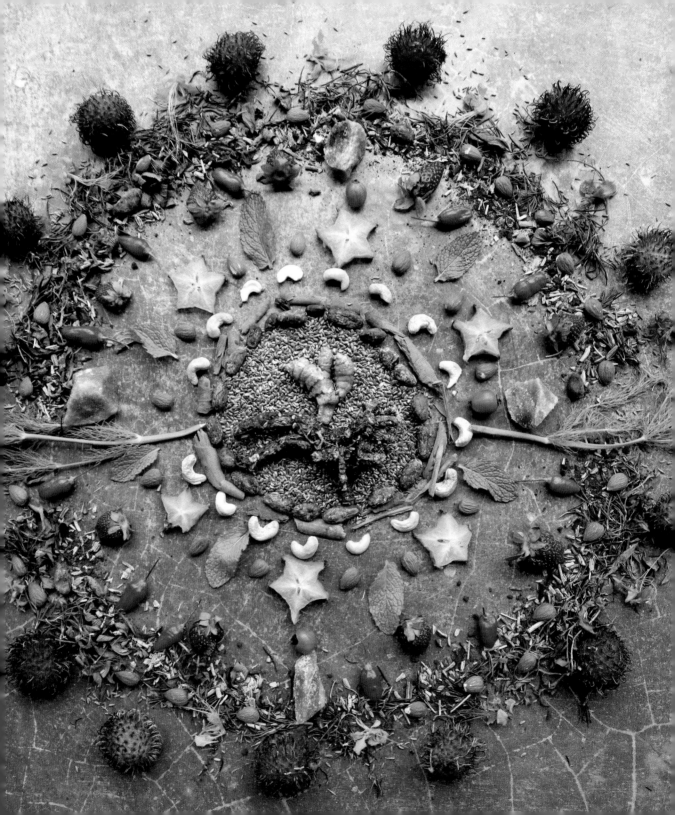

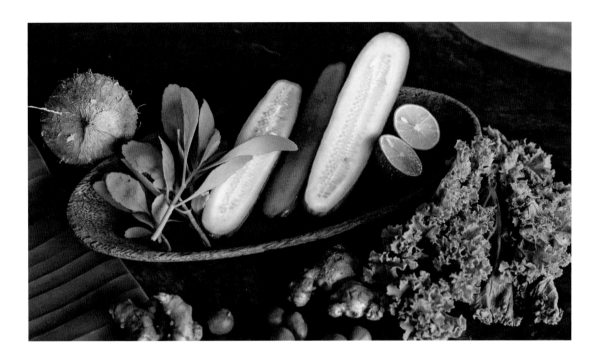

We are at a time of remarkable abundance, and now, due to technology, we have access to the rarest and most powerful herbs nature has to offer. Perhaps it's the first time in human history that we are experiencing access to the most healing herbs and foods from all over the world. Even though our problems as a society can seem overwhelming, we are still making progress as a global community in becoming more self-aware, spiritually oriented, and healthier overall. We truly are becoming a whole other class of humans due to having access to ancient knowledge and maximum nutritional availability through miraculous herbs and foods.

SUPERFOODS

A superfood is both a food and a medicine with a remarkably potent and supernutrient-rich chemistry. It is more potent than regular food due to its ability to immediately increase vital force and energy in the body. Superfoods are tasty and grounding, and provide essential nutrition to major organ systems. A superfood's potent and concentrated chemistry exceeds daily nutritional requirements in certain areas, such as vitamin, mineral, and protein content. Superfoods nourish us at a cellular level, fueling our entire body with vibrant power.

Superfoods have demonstrated the ability to gently bring the body back to alignment, supporting restoration to its original constitution. Superfoods can take charge and keep the body in balance by regulating blood sugar for a longer time, making sure we have enough mineral storage in the body, and maintaining ongoing detoxification. Scientists have yet to discover all the nutrients found within plants. In fact, there are so many available and yet-to-be discovered nutrients in regularly used plants that we are receiving innumerable additional benefits that we've yet to understand!

Due to the depletion of nutrients in conventional foods, even within mass organic plantations, we've had to continue to turn to new possibilities to live a truly wholesome and balanced life. Superfoods have contributed to this global issue by providing a medium to receive the higher-level nutritive power that our body demands as a basic right. Therefore, now that superfoods are available even in regular grocery stores, we need to turn to the next level to receive balance.

SUPERHERBS

The miraculous group of botanicals commonly referred to as tonic superherbs are medicinal products that can be consumed daily with foods. Out of the 40,000 herbs worldwide, about 80 of them are tonic herbs. Tonic herbs are adaptogenic, meaning they are remarkable botanicals that help the body adapt to stress, support metabolic functions, and restore balance. They are powerful sources known to increase the body's resistance to physical, biological, emotional, and environmental stressors and provide a defense response to acute or chronic stress. They are a particular category of herbs known to restore endocrine hormones (which includes the adrenals, thyroid, parathyroid, pituitary gland, pancreas, and reproductive organs), and that also modulate the immune system and allow the body to maintain optimal homeostasis.

The awesome power of superherbs lies in their ability to be friendly to most body types and their ability to teach the body to remain at balance. They are potent movers and shakers in the body, yet they produce minimal (or no) side effects on physical or mental health. Depending on the category of herbs used, some don't require as much care in exact dosing as others. For example, adaptogens are master tonic herbs that regulate body systems through cellular balancing and maintaining positive homeostasis.. These herbs require careful dosage. Some adaptogens are reishi, chaga, and schisandra berries. On the other hand, the category of herbs known as nervines support the nervous system. These herbs have a range of effects and can be mildly calm-

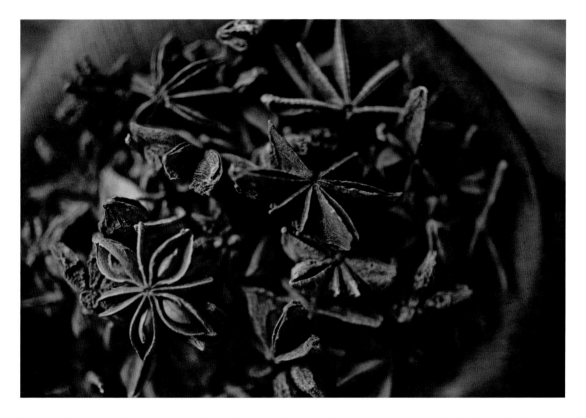

ing, anti-spasmodic, or strongly sedative. A few nerving herbs are passionflower, mimosa, and valerian. In very high doses or in combination with certain pharmaceuticals, however, they can cause some unwanted side effects.

The awesome power of superherbs lies in their ability to be friendly to most body types and their ability to teach the body to remain at balance. Many tonic herbs have high anti-oxidant properties similar to many superfoods, as well as a wide range of healing abilities, and can even support multiple systems. These miraculous herbs have been known to operate on multiple levels to bring back equilibrium in the body and mind.

SUPERHERBS: HERBAL TONICS

5

What Is an Herbal Tonic?

Herbal tonics are a potent selection of herbs known to deeply restore, tone, and invigorate multiple body systems. An herbal tonic is a solution or preparation of one or many herbs known to holistically promote health, and be a medicinal source to the mind, body, and spirit.

Many would say that most herbs are tonics. For an herb to be recognized as a tonic, the herb must have been found over many centuries of human use and study to meet specific qualifications. Tonic herbs are said to provide "adaptive energy," which helps us handle stress much more easily. It is possible to develop a very high degree of adaptability to the many challenges we face and the changes that constantly take place in our lives. By overcoming stressful circumstances successfully, we grow as human beings and we enjoy life much more fully and with radiance. The superior herbs are thus a primary source of true human empowerment.

A few keys to knowing about tonic herbs:

- A tonic herb must have anti-aging properties, meaning it is known to support a healthy and long life free of disease.
- A tonic herb must have a profound health-promoting chemistry that produces noticeable positive health effects within a short period of time after consumption.
- Tonics must help balance physical, emotional, and psychic energy—so as to truly improve one's spiritual well-being and happiness.
- Tonic herbs are known to not have side effects—they are meant to be used

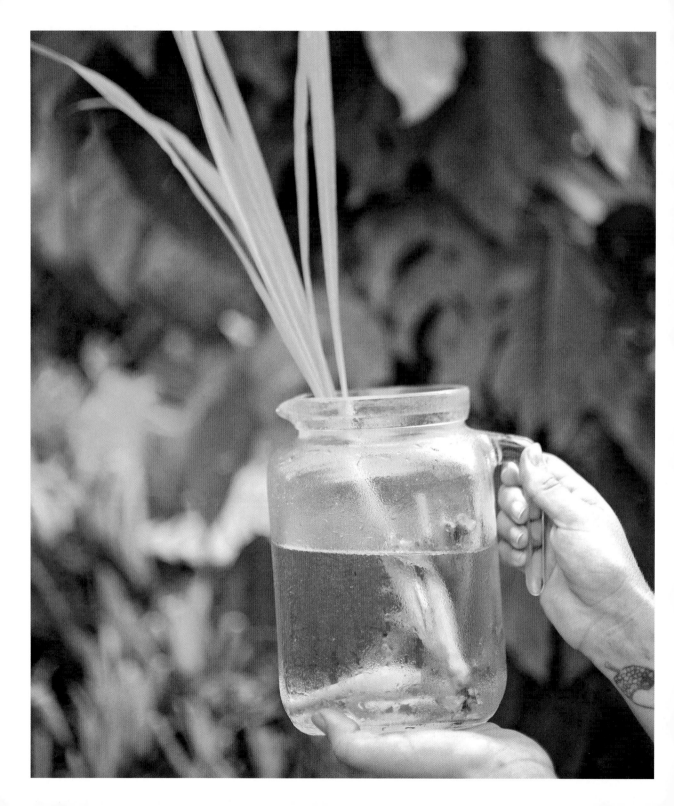

over a long time in order for the body to take in long-term benefits. In fact, tonic herbs are known to be gentle and friendly herbs that most, if not all, people can take with no severe effects.

- Most tonic herbs are like foods— they tend to be easily digestible and assimilable; you can add them to your food and drink, enhancing the flavor and effects of any carrier you choose.

Basically, herbal tonics are by definition herbs that safely promote one's health and healthy aging through regular consumption. Tonics are particularly effective because they "teach" the body over time, creating positive effects that eventually operate in the body without the assistance of the tonic. To this day, more and more studies are uncovering the existence of tonic herbs and demonstrating the chemical response they generate in the body over time.

Nowadays, tonic herbs grow in many places throughout the world (China, the Himalayas, Mongolia, Central Asia, Southeast Asia, India, Indonesia, Africa, South America, North America, Europe, and Oceania). But, the principles of tonic herbalism were established by the ancients in Asia, particularly by great Daoist teachers: Asian wise men and women. These principles are profound and

time tested, and are now largely supported by modern science and modern theories of health and healthy aging.

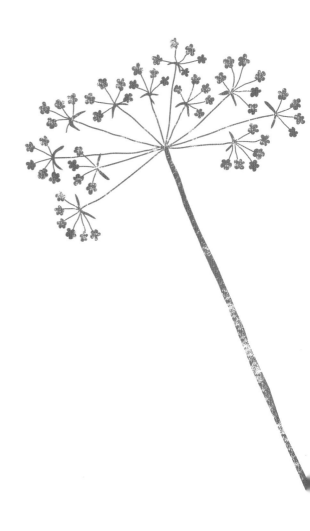

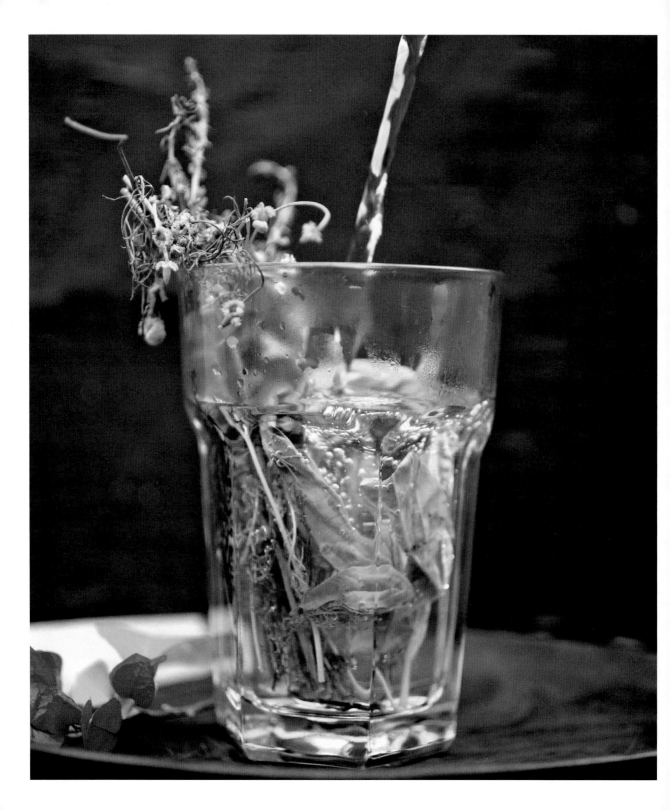

6

Basic Techniques for Creating Herbal Tonics

Often, the best medicines are those we make ourselves. While paying for the convenience of having someone make it for us, prepackaged products are just that: put together outside the realm of our control, from components with which we may not be entirely familiar. Tonics made with our own hands can be carefully constructed. We can be empowered by the knowledge that we have chosen each ingredient and have controlled the process of producing them. Tonics can be made in a wide variety of ways. Each root, mushroom, bark, leaf, and flower is best extracted using a specific process. According to the chemistry it carries and the amount of water it naturally contains, you can decide on the optimal form in which to receive the entire benefits of your formula.

THE ELEMENTS OF MAKING HERBAL TONICS AND ELIXIRS

Regardless of what form you choose, you will always get some benefit regardless of your process. Even if an herb is used in an infusion, making an extract out of it is still a fantastic option!

Tea

Vehicle: hot water.

How to Make an Infusion

I recommend making infusions with leaves and flowers.

- Add fresh or dry herbs to a teapot.
- Add hot (almost boiling) water to the herbs.
- Steep for 5–10 minutes.

How to Make a Decoction

I recommend making decoctions with roots, mushrooms, barks, and stems. But some herbs also require simmering in order to fully extract a particular chemistry.

- Add your ingredients into a pot (ideally ceramic or stainless steel).
- The basic proportion for a decoction is 1 part water and 1 part of root or herb.
- Simmer for about 20–30 minutes with the lid off until the volume of water is reduced by one quarter.
- Strain and enjoy.
- Decoctions can be stored in the fridge for up to 3 days.

Liquid Extracts

The best vehicles for liquid extracts are alcohol, vinegar, and vegetable glycerin.

How to Make an Extract with Alcohol

- Use a strong grain alcohol or vodka (no less than 25% [50 proof]).
- A good ratio for dried plant material is about 1 part herbs to 5 parts alcohol.
- A good ratio for fresh plant material is 1 part herbs to 3 parts alcohol.
- Keep in mind that for fresh plant extract you must use a higher percentage of alcohol—at least 40% (80 proof).
- If using fresh herbs, chop the herbs finely.
- Add the herbs to a clean jar, and fill up with the alcohol all the way until covering the herbs.
- After adding the alcohol, place plastic wrap over the mouth of the jar and cover with a tight-fitting lid, sandwiching the wrap between the lid and the jar. This will prevent rust and contamination.
- Shake well, and allow the herbs to set for 3–4 weeks. This allows at least a whole lunar cycle, which is known to be just the right amount of time to extract

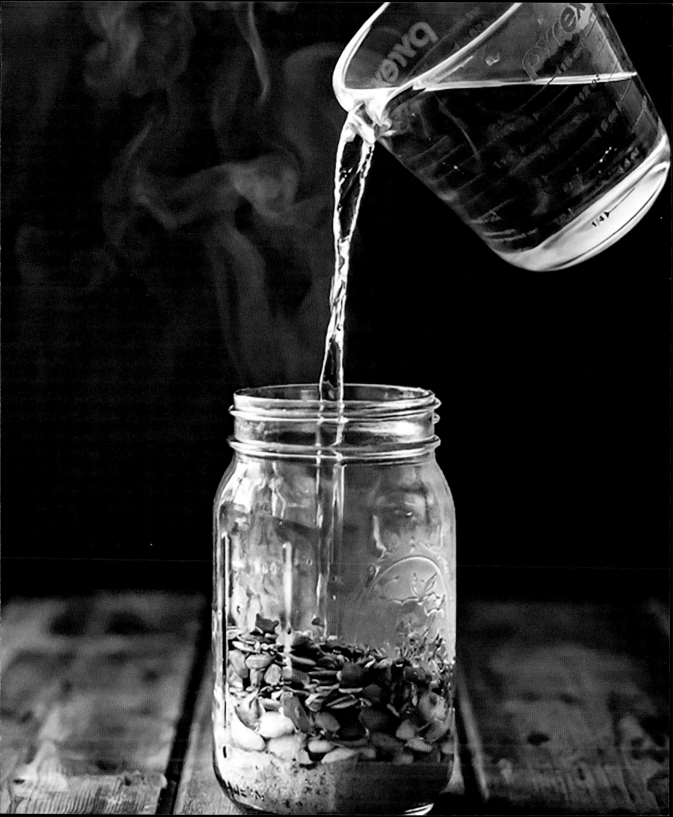

the necessary chemistry out of the herb.

- Shake every other day. The movement helps the herbs loosen and release.
- Strain the herbs out with a mesh cloth (any fine cloth or cheesecloth works as well), and press the liquid out.
- Funnel the liquid into an amber or blue bottle and store in a cool dark place.
- Voilà! You have now made a potent medicinal extract. The amount you made will last you quite some time, and it will keep for up to 5 years.

How to Make an Extract with Vegetable Glycerin

Sometimes referred to as glycerol, glycerin is a clear, colorless, and odorless liquid with an incredibly sweet taste that has the consistency of thick syrup. Glycerin has been used as an ingredient in toothpaste, shampoos, soaps, herbal remedies, and other household items.

- Fill a jar halfway with dried herbs (two-thirds full with fresh herbs)
- In a separate container mix 3 parts vegetable glycerin and 1 part filtered water. Mix well to combine.
- Pour the liquid mixture over the herb, and completely cover to fill the jar.
- Shake daily or every other day to loosen the herbs and help them extract better.

- Allow to steep for 4–6 weeks.
- Strain with cheesecloth, and press the herbs until they are dry.
- Pour the liquid into an amber or blue bottle, and voilà! You have made a potent and medicinal glycerin!

How to Make an Extract with Vinegar

- Fill a clean jar about halfway with dried herbs.
- Pour apple cider vinegar over the herbs until the jar is filled to the top.
- Place plastic wrap over the mouth of the jar, and cover with a tight-fitting lid, sandwiching the wrap between the lid and the jar to prevent rusting.
- Allow to extract for 14 days in a cool, dark place.
- Shake daily or every other day to ensure the herbs are loosened.
- Strain with a mesh cloth, and funnel into a glass bottle.
- You can drink the vinegar directly or use it for cooking for an extra delicious and medicinal touch.

JUICE COCKTAILS: JUICE TONICS

The Anatomy of a Superherb Tonic

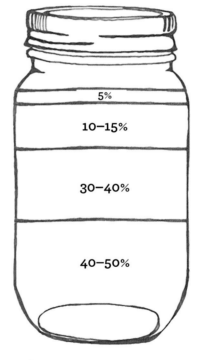

4. Mother Extract
   5%
3. Infusions & Decoctions
   10–15%
2. Fruits & Roots Juice
   30–40%
1. Veggie & Herb Juice
   40–50%

1. **Veggies:** Make about 40–50% of your juice to be veggies, greens, and fresh herbs. A mix of cold-pressed greens (dark leafy greens, parsley, dandelion, spinach, broccoli, cucumber, celery, etc)
2. **Fruit or Roots:** Make 30—40% of your juice be fruits and roots. A mix of cold-pressed fruits, (apple, pear, coconut, pinespple, dragon fruit, citrus, beets, carrots, etc.).
3. **Infusions:** Make 10–15% of the juice be your herbal infusion/decoction concentrate. An infused mix of leaves, barks and flowers (chamomile, roses, horsetail, pau d'arco, mushrooms, etc.)
4. **Mother Extract:** Make 5% of your juice be your herbal extract. As the finishing touch, add 1 tablespoon of your herbal tonic (mother extract) to your juice.

Techniques for Juicing with Superherbs

If you want to create healthy and delicious cold-pressed juices, of course having the best juicer for your home kitchen is the best option. If you aren't ready to make that investment, there are other routes to having cold-pressed magic in your kitchen. Cold-pressing is a great process for juicing because the bio-active and enzyme quality of the juice it produces is maintained by pressing with no heat. Regardless of the machine you have on hand, keep in mind that the most important aspect of preserving the nutritional integrity of your juice is no heat and slow juicing.

JUICER OPTIONS FOR HOME

Cold-pressing juicers and slow masticating juicers are the absolute best ways to produce juices with a variety of nutritional benefits. There are quite a few options on the market. Just be sure to buy slow masticating juicers, as opposed to the ones that run hot and fast and tend to burn the juice within a minute after you first begin juicing. You can tell if your juicer is a good one by how the pulp comes out. If it comes out very dry, it means your juicer is using a lot more fiber per liquid ounce. If it's mushy and wet, the machine rushed through the juicing process and didn't masticate efficiently enough. If this is the case, always be sure to hand-press your pulp to get the nutritious cold-press aspect to your juice.

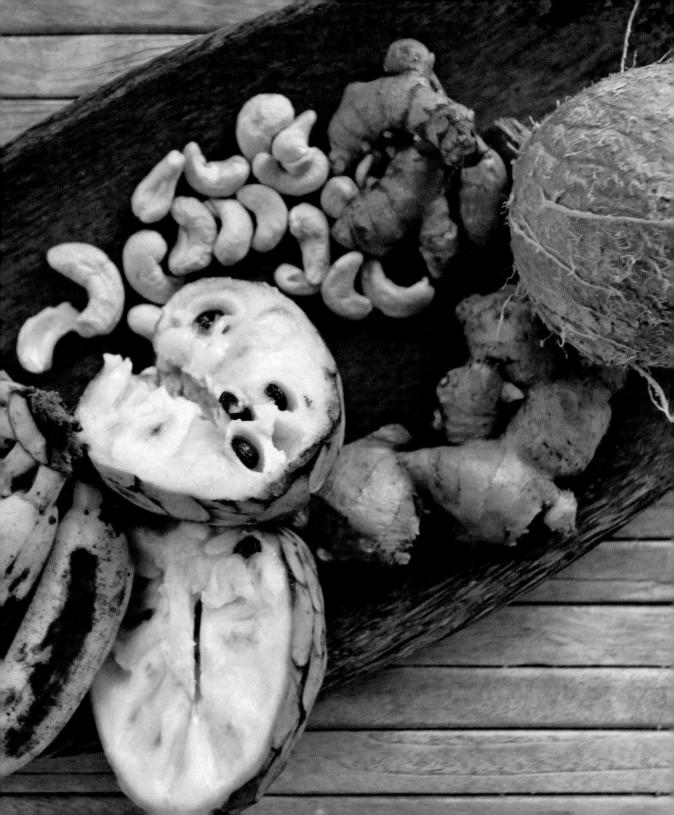

Here are some of my favorite juicers:

Norwalk®: These machines can be quite an investment, but they are fantastic if you are looking to take juicing to the next level. The Norwalk has a non-heat-induced masticator, with a side compartment where you press the juice in a bag. A lot of people love this, but also it takes a lot of time (and cleaning!) to use.

Champion®: My personal favorite. The juice quality it produces is silky and delicious, and there are many options in terms of the masticator. You can buy separate compartments for milling wheatgrass, making gelato at home, and more. The Champion is more affordable than many other options and easy to use. I still recommend saving the pulp and hand-pressing it to get the best part of the juice out.

Omega 8006/8005/8004 Masticating Juicers®: The pulp from these machines is the driest I have seen. That means maximum nutrition, and you'll also like how it breaks down into four easy-to-clean parts.

MASTICATING JUICERS & CENTRIFUGAL JUICERS

Masticating juicers are higher-end machines with a price range from $250 to $500. They are worth the investment. Centrifugal juicers are priced from $100 to $300. Always choose the masticating variety, if possible, to ensure a longer-lasting machine and better-quality juice.

Follow these basic rules to get silky cold-press juice from most machines:

Go slowly: Don't overheat the engine. Have the machine slowly chew down the ingredients.

Your pulp is holy: Run your pulp through the masticator again to press all the necessary nutrients out, or simply press by hand using cheesecloth. Even if you are just using a blender to make a juice (not a smoothie), use a fine-mesh cloth, and filter out all the extra fiber to get an exquisite silky juice.

HOMEMADE HYDRAULIC PRESS

If you're someone who likes to get crafty or have something utilitarian around, homemade hydraulic presses are fantastic. Before juicers were made, this was the technology most people all over the world used to be able to manually press or lift tons of weight without a lot of physical labor. Indigenous peoples used the hydraulic press for a variety of things; for example, in the rainforest, huge hydraulic presses were used to make cane juice. The press would exude about 10 tons of power with a simple rotating device to squeeze out every possible ounce of liquid.

BLENDERS & HAND FILTRATION

Blenders are not really for making juice, yet they can play a key role in providing healthy juice if this is all you have. Blending gives you either a pulpier juice or a smoothie. Sometimes when I'm traveling and I don't have anything but a blender, I make juice with it. Cold-press snobs would probably disapprove, but this is how to make magic with whatever you have. For example, to make watermelon juice, blend it on low speed (to keep it raw and unoxidized), leave it a bit pulpy and chunky, pour it into a fine-mesh cloth, and carefully press out the juice. That's it! Easy. If you want a juice with less fiber, keep filtering—although you might be surprised to find that by a third filtration you still get little pieces of pulp.

Basically, treat the blender as a masticator, and hand-press the juice after blending to filter out the pulp. Again, although the end result is not cold-pressed juice, if you are in a pinch or traveling, a blender can be your savior!

ADDING TONIC HERBS TO YOUR JUICE

Once the fresh juice is ready, add your tonic herbs. Several ways you can make medicines have been covered, but here are all the ways you can easily add the medicine to the juice.

HERBAL CONCENTRATES

Certain herbs are best to have stocked in the fridge as a liquid concentrate. For example, your decoctions of barks, roots, leaves, or mushrooms are best stored in the fridge after boiling them for several hours. This way, you can keep an ongoing stock that lasts you up to three days. Herbal concentrates naturally get better the more they sit, and many alkaloids and other chemical constituents release only after a few hours of being cooked down.

Once the veggie and fruit juice is ready, the general rule of thumb is to add about 1 to 2 ounces of liquid herbal concentrate to the juice (for a 14- to 16-ounce glass). If you start venturing out of your comfort zone and begin using other herbs, make sure you're familiar with the herb you are using so you can adjust the dosage. You don't want to overdo it.

TONICS & ELIXIRS

These are all the tonics you've made or bought that are extracted in alcohol, vegetable glycerin, or vinegar. For extracts, depending on strength, add ½ to 1 teaspoon to your juice in a 14- to 16-ounce glass.

POWDERED HERBS

I love using shakers. For powdered herbs, a good ratio is 1 teaspoon per 16 ounces of juice. Add to a classic shaker or shake it in a glass jar.

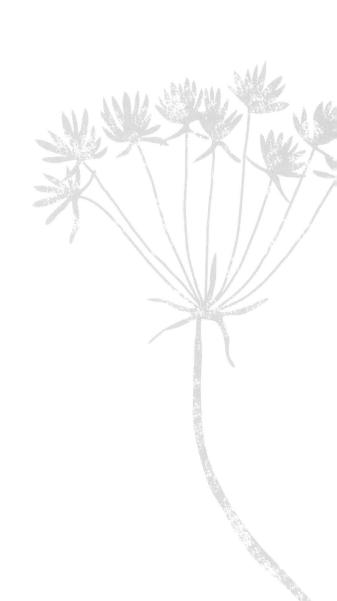

9

Top 20 Must-Haves for Every Kitchen

It's hard to condense a list of essentials and favorites. Usually my kitchen is stocked with all kinds of weeds, roots, and barks, having more than a hundred different kinds of beautiful botanicals. I recommend that people not get overwhelmed with overstocking the kitchen with too many unfamiliar herbs. It's good to start off with a seasonal selection of essentials and slowly start building from there, familiarizing with different botanicals. When you go on a walk, be on the lookout for your favorite herbs—they are some of the healthiest and most vibrant forms of medicine readily available.

This list contains essential herbal staples I love that grow all over the world. It covers the major and minor necessities we have on a regular and seasonal basis for optimum wellness.

TOP 20 MUST-HAVES

These are the herbal tonics that I cannot live without. Within these 20 you find all the basic essentials you possibly need within a home pharmacy—immunity booster, beauty, vitamin C, colds and flus, bones and muscle health, digestive health, weight loss, and so on.

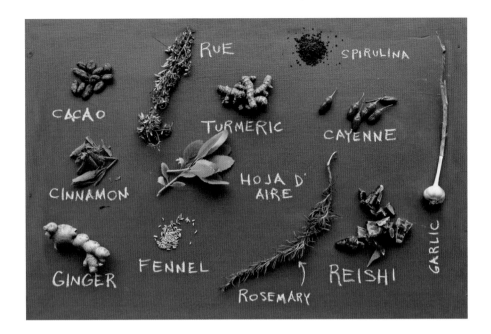

1. Graviola (Annona muricata)

Graviola is a rainforest essential known to be a potent antibacterial, antimicrobial, antiparasitic, antitumoral, anticancer powerhouse. Annonaceous acetogenins are only found in the Annonaceae family (to which graviola belongs). These chemicals in general have been documented with antitumorous, antiparasitic, insecticidal, and antimicrobial activities. Many studies have recently determined that these acetogenins are superb inhibitors of enzyme processes that are found only in the membranes of cancerous tumor cells. This is why they are toxic to cancer cells but have no toxicity to healthy cells.

2. Moringa (Moringa oleifera)

Moringa is a miracle tree known to contain a megaload of antioxidants, minerals, protein, essential fiber, and cleansing properties. Also known for its power to supply sustainable energy, lower blood pressure, and aid in adrenal support, moringa acts as a coagulant, attaching itself to harmful material and toxins within the body and flushing them quite rapidly.

3. Jergón Sacha (Dracontium loretense)

Jergón sacha is a signature plant of the Amazon, containing some of the most potent antiviral chemistry found in nature. Indian tribes throughout the Amazon rainforest use the large tuber or rhizome of the jergón sacha plant as an antidote for the bite of snakes. It has also been used to treat bites from spiders, stingrays, and other poisonous animals. It makes a potent antibacterial, antimicrobial, and anticancer tonic, and supports healing from radiation as well as genital diseases.

4. Suma (Pfaffia paniculata)

Suma is also referred to as "Brazilian ginseng" and is known as a master tonic and adaptogen found in the Amazon. The benefits of suma are astonishingly similar to those of regular ginsengs. It has been used for generations as a general cure-all, and has served as everything from an energy and vitality tonic to cellular oxygenator, appetite stimulant, anti-inflammatory and circulatory medicine, blood sugar balancer, and most popularly an immune booster.

5. Chanca Piedra (Phyllantus niruri)

Chanca piedra is referred to as the "stone-breaker" and is also known as the rainforest's most potent liver and gall bladder detoxifer. It was named for its effective use by generations of Amazonian indigenous peoples in eliminating gallstones and kidney stones. It is a super tonic with long-documented use to support treatment of hepatitis, colds and flus, tuberculosis, liver diseases and disorders, anemia, and liver cancer.

6. Turmeric (Curcuma longa)

Turmeric is an anti-inflammatory and vitamin C tonic root. It is a great daily remedy to keep inflammation at bay by alkalizing and soothing the digestive system and the liver. It This masterful tonic for joints, muscles, soft tissue, and skin generates strength and elasticity and is a fantastic anti-aging root.

7. Tulsi (Ocimum tenuiflorum)

Tulsi is Ayurveda's holiest of herbs, an adaptogenic powerhouse known for its digestive healing abilities, cardiovascular protection, and potent anti-inflammatory nature. It lowers cholesterol levels, prevents hypoglycemia, eases stress by calming the nervous system, prevents migraines, and repairs skin damage (topically and internally). It is a great overall superherb.

8. Nettle (Urtica dioica)

Nettle is an excellent daily remedy for overall longevity known for its anti-inflammatory, bone-building, blood-nourishing, testosterone-building, silica-gifting superherb qualities. The leaves and the seeds are also used in nerve repair and as a central nervous system regulator. The roots are usually used for testosterone- and prostate-building qualities, yet it's also a great energizer that all can benefit from—not just men. It's a wonderful tea to have, and it can be combined with other tonics to enhance its qualities.

9. Reishi (*Ganoderma lucidum*)
Research on the chemistry and therapeutic benefits of mushrooms like reishi have been extensive for centuries. Reishi is an immune modulator capable of restoring the immune system and is often used for therapies before and after cancer. The polysaccharides present within the mushrooms are extraordinary cancer-fighting compounds. This amazing mushroom is known as a supreme lung and cardio tonic, supportive in lowering bad cholesterol and triglycerides.

10. Chaga (*Inonotus obliquus*)
Chaga is the master tonic for the immune system. It supports the elimination of tumors, cancerous cells, autoimmune diseases, and environmental traumas (such as radiation, pollution, heavy metals, etc.)

11. Pau D'Arco (*Tabebuia impetiginosa*)
This sacred pau d'arco tree has been worshipped for hundreds of years, and its bark has been used as an antifungal and anti-inflammatory. It is used traditionally for blood sugar and blood pressure imbalances, ulcers, digestive imbalances, parasites, yeast infections, cancer, diabetes, and allergies.

12. Sangre de Drago (*Croton lechleri*)
Sangre de drago is claimed to be the best wound healer in nature. It is a tree known to bleed a miracle resin when you slice off some of the bark. This thick red resin is known to act as a potent internal and external bandage with intensive antibiotic support. Also known for its powerful antiseptic qualities, it has a potent antiviral and antimicrobial ability. Many have also used it as an anticancerous support as well as for healing from radiation.

13. Cat's Claw (*Unicaria tomentosa*)
Cat's claw is known as the master immune booster of the Amazon. It is one of the oldest herbs with recorded history in the rainforest, noted for its immune-modulating power and anticancer, antirheumatic, and anti-arthritic properties.

14. Ginseng (*Panax ginseng*)
A superior tonic remedy, ginseng has been regarded for centuries as the king of medicinal herbs. In Chinese medicine, not only is it regarded an adaptogen and energizer, it's also used to calm the spirit, eliminate anxious and stressed *qi* (energy), open the heart, and strengthen the mind. Asian and American ginseng have both been used to strengthen the heart, spleen, lungs, liver, and kidneys.

15. Spirulina (Anthrospira platensis)

Known as the world's highest source of complete protein (around 65% by weight), spirulina, or blue-green algae, provides a vast array of trace elements and macrominerals. Blue-green algae is a wild-grown superfood that also contains plenty of phytonutrients and enzymes.

16. Horsetail (Equisetum arvense)

Horsetail is one of the most ancient plants in nature. Known for its excellent ability to heal bones, bone marrow, and wounds in general thanks to its high silica content, it contains high amounts of calcium as well as silica in minerals that specialize in repairing connective tissue, bone alignment and healing, and skin repair. It is also used for the kidneys, eyes, and hair, and for immune regulation.

17. Rhodiola (Rhodiola rosea)

Rhodiola is a magical root known to strengthen the nervous system, fight depression, enhance immunity and memory, aid weight loss, increase sexual function, and improve energy levels. It has been effectively used to prevent depression and to support post-traumatic stress disorder. It enhances the transport of serotonin precursors, tryptophan, and 5-hydroxytryptophan into the brain.

18. Mangosteen (Garcinia mangostana)

Mangosteen is queen of the tropical fruits. Not only is it a delicious fruit, but the peel of the mangosteen is perhaps one of the most loaded vitamin C sources ever known. It contains a huge amount of antioxidants known for their anti-aging and longevity attributes. It is also a master tonic for the endocrine and immune systems, is known to support healing of wounds and damaged nerves, and can assist in weight loss.

19. Gynostemma (Gynostemma pentaphyllum)

Also known as jiaogulan, gynostemma is an adaptogen and antioxidant with chemical constituents similar to ginseng. The leaf is known for its ability to lower blood pressure, purify the blood, support the pancreas, and release stress out of the body, and it can support weight loss by assisting in the metabolism of fats.

20. Schisandra Berries (Schisandra chinensis)

Schisandra berries are one of the few botanical sources containing all five flavors: sweet,, sour, salty, bitter, and pungent. These super-berries are known to be adaptogens, liver protectors, blood purifiers and nourishers, and master tonic to the five organs. Among many more healing benefits, the master tonic made from these berries prevents fatigue and boosts the body with endurance and strength.

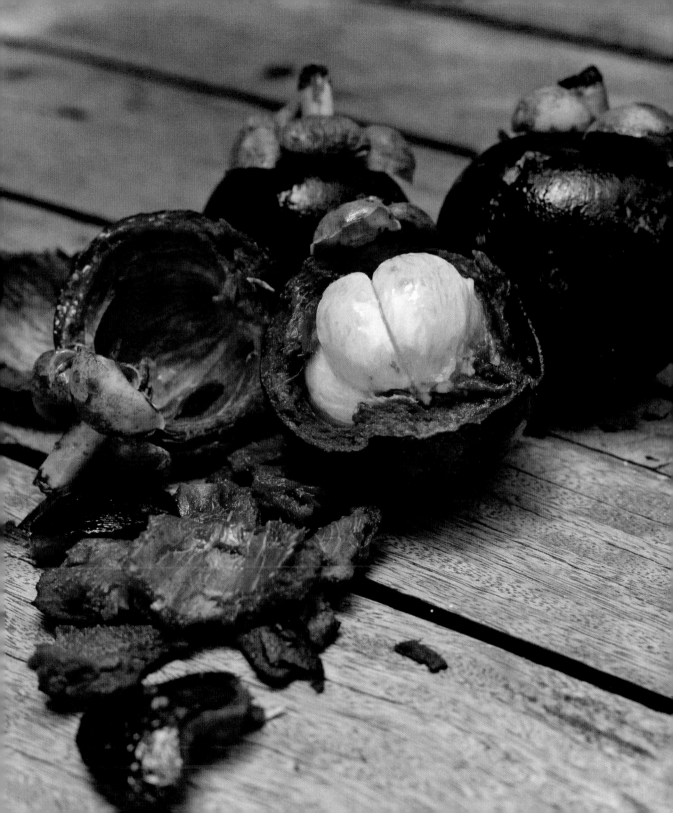

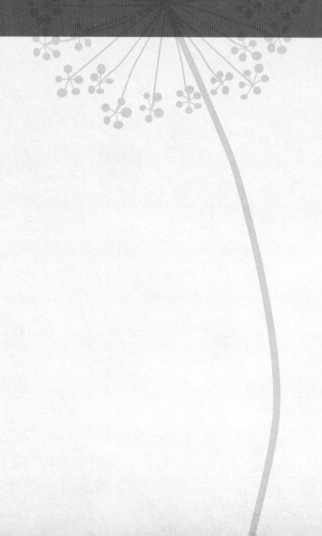

JUICING THE RAINBOW

10

The Rainbow Diet

The key to creating the optimal diet for yourself is to understand that there is no single best diet for everyone. Every single person is a biochemical universe within him- or herself, composed of physical, emotional, and spiritual history. Human DNA has millions of variations, and most of the human body is still an undiscovered landscape by modern science. It is not surprising that those of us living within a human condition should have least several different basic diets to choose among, according to our genetic physiology. Knowing these facts, how can we possibly try to fit a single diet or supplement regime that works for everyone and every disease?

Whether you eat macrobiotic, paleo, raw, vegan, low-protein vegetarian, high-protein, or low-fat and high-carbohydrate—all of these options usually are only compatible with about one-third of their participants. This doesn't mean the diet doesn't work; it simply means that some constitutions will resonate with a particular regime, whereas others won't.

Our body clock is precisely timed with the seasons, the weather, the moon, and planetary movements. The more we can stay local and in tune with the current season, the more the body will thrive. It is of utmost importance to pay attention daily to what you want and need rather than sticking to a philosophy that doesn't necessarily resonate with you within the different cycles of life.

The rainbow diet is a base from which to work. From this base, you can build in accordance to whatever season your body is in. By committing to these basic principles, you can flourish organically and monitor your wellness by intuitively listening to your body's needs. These basic principles act as longevity staples for any time:

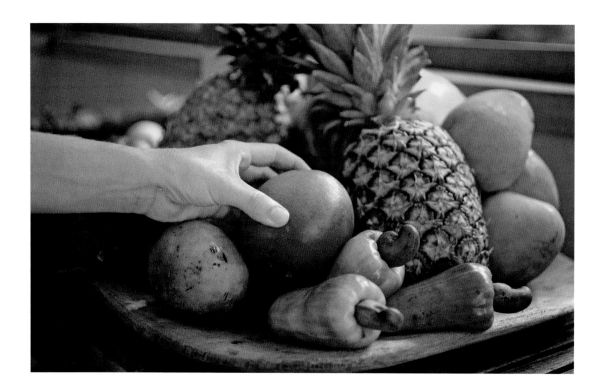

1. Eat vibrant, fresh foods.

2. Eat with the seasons.

3. Have most, if not all, of the rainbow colors present at every meal.

4. Integrate tonic superherbs in between meals.

5. Create a peaceful internal environment every time you sit down to eat.

Keeping these five basic intentions intact will provide a longevity base for you to work with. Ayurveda, Tibetan medicine, and Chinese medicine share similar constitutional theories with respect to creating a healing cosmology.

The rainbow diet takes elemental body types that occur in many different ancient healing traditions into account: Earth, Fire, and Air/Water. We will review the different body types in the next chapter. Ancient traditions hold that our basic constitutions fall into one of several general patterns within the millions of kinds of bodies on our planet, shifting in tune with seasonal rhythms and phases of life, as well as the cycles and rhythms of the planet.

11

Medicines for Your Body Type

The human body is like Mother Earth. A perfect synergy of elements is constantly in play to keep a biochemical and homeostatic balance. Through the astute balance of these internal elementals, we achieve longevity and harmony. We must keep in mind how all the archetypes of the universe reside within our body and mind. These constitutional theories are recorded maps of human patterning that help us understand the ins and outs of the body's cycles. We all contain each body type to a certain degree; it's more of a matter of understanding where we are at a given time and how we can achieve a greater balance through diet, tonic herbs, daily practice, and emotional awakening.

I've broken down the elemental body constitutions into three main body types. Each body type is an integration of several traditions: Ayurveda, traditional Chinese medicine (TCM), Mayan, and medical astrology.

EARTH BODY

Energetics: Moist, wet, oily, hot, sticky

Body Components: Stomach, intestines, digestive tract

Chakra: Base, sacral

Ayurveda: Kapha

on September 22, is the equinox day, first day, usu
darkness finally equals   when nights
After this,   the length of the day
me longer   the nights
ntil   than
er   the
he   Sol
ight,   lon
hese   Dec
easonal   day
round   cha
ex   the
erfect   are
leanse   tim
nd   the
the Self   Rig
work.   for

Autumn

		ELEMENT		
DIRECTION	METAL		COLOR	
WEST			WHITE	
CLIMATE DRY			QUALITY HARVEST	
EMOTION WORRY GRIEF			SENSE/ORGAN NOSE SMELL	
SOUND WEEP			FLUID MUCUS	
TASTE PUNGENT			INDICATOR BODY HAIR	
SMELL ROTTEN	LUNGS	LARGE INTESTINE	SKIN—HAIR TISSUE	

YIN — ORGANS — YANG

in-balance	*imbalance*
consolidation	indecision
communication	confusion
new disciplines—productive work	overindulgence
study, clarity, care	coffee, smoking
quiet walks	obscurity
more rest	fatigue

The
eginning
f the
ARK,
in
cycle

Metal Element

- TCM: Earth/Water
- Astrological Rulers: Saturn, Venus, Moon

This body type is blessed with endurance, strength, and stamina. The Earth body types are grounded and stable, constantly seeking that which is at ease, comfortable, and harmonic. When Earth types are in balance, they are the sweetest of people, with gentle auras and a stabilizing presence. Naturally, Earth types have a slower metabolism and have a thicker build, but only when out of balance do they start collecting belly fat. This body type tends to carry all of the weight around the belly, keeping slender arms and legs.

If they are out of balance, even if it's for a short phase, they must keep in mind that this type of energy is what brings diseases into fruition quite quickly.

The Earth body psychology tends to be very patient, calm, tolerant, and forgiving. However, it does tend to get sluggish, lazy, and lethargic if it is not in alignment. Out of balance, feelings of possession, attachment, greed, and envy may surge.

The Earth body naturally stores energy, so it must be a number one priority to keep diseases at bay. The Water principle within Earth allows for certain climate conditions to manifest, for example, water retention, sinus congestion, inflamed mucous membranes, toxic accumulation within fat tissue, diabetes, and so on.

COMMON CRAVINGS: Sweet, salty, starchy, oily foods

BALANCED CRAVINGS: Bitter, astringent, pungent

Response to a poor diet: Lethargic, lack of energy, ongoing cravings

Therapeutic foods: Plenty of leafy greens (kale, collards, chard, spinach, romaine), light proteins (legumes, seaweed, fish) supplemented with healthy fats (avocado, nuts, seeds, nut butter, coconut oil, olive oil, full-fat cheeses, eggs). Very low doses of raw oils (raw coconut oil, flax seed, borage oil). Low doses of honey and yacon as sweeteners.

Therapeutic herbs: Bitters!* Dandelion leaf and root, quassia bark, orange peel, Oregon grape root, mustard leaf and seed, mugwort, rue, milk thistle, burdock root, yarrow, cardamom, yellow dock

---

* Bitters are particularly beneficial because they will accelerate Earth's metabolism while repairing the gut to digest better.

Other healing tonics: Alfalfa, blackberry leaf, chamomile, cinnamon, cleavers, ginger, hawthorn, hyssop, lemon, nettle, parsley seed and leaf, skullcap, spearmint, thyme, wild carrot

Limit: Starchy carbs and low–glycemic index fruits (berries) to one meal a day.

Must eliminate: Sugary refined carbohydrates (like sports drinks), dense foods like store-bought energy bars or "health" drinks, products that have a yogurt-like consistency. Stay away from dairy! Dairy ferments quite quickly in the gut, and within a low metabolism it generates quite a lot of inflammation.

Lucky you: Dominant Earth types tend to get away with the occasional use of coffee and other stimulants, as well as with the occasional glass of wine.

FIRE BODY

Energetics: Warm, hot, oily

Body Components: Intestines, diaphragm

Chakra: Solar plexus, heart

Ayurveda: Kapha

TCM: Earth/Water

Astrological Rulers: Mars, Sun, Jupiter

Fire types are penetrating, hot, and sharp people. They tend to have a nice build, medium height, and coppery skin, with a constant warm body (perhaps even sweating constantly). Their hair tends to be silky and at times tends to gray faster than others' due to all the energy they burn. Fire body types are lucky to have a strong metabolism with overall good digestion and a big appetite. They tend to be constantly alert, with a sharp mind and usually with good powers of comprehension. Naturally, fire types are good leaders and planners, constantly desiring to work with the community and alleviate problems around them.

Fire body types need to be careful with inflammation, whether it be fevers, skin disorders, or inflammatory diseases in any organ. They must also take care not to bottle up emotions or generate deep discomfort toward situations in life. This tends to generate emotional imbalance or a type of inflammation related to it, like ulcers and other digestive issues.

COMMON CRAVINGS: Spicy, hot, sour, salty

BALANCED CRAVINGS: Sweet, bitter, astringent

Response to a poor diet: Anxiety, anger, hypoglycemia, acid reflux

Therapeutic foods: All grains (particularly amaranth, barley, rice oats), vegetables, and raw foods really calm the fire down. A wholesale macro-type diet keeps the fire at bay. Nuts and raw oils are good in moderation (particularly coconut oil, almond oil, sesame oil, and flax oil). Seeds are more beneficial due to low oil content. Beans (particularly chickpeas, mung beans, adzuki beans, and black lentils) are a good source of light protein and are easily digestible without generating too much heat. Dark leafy greens are always a substantial and cooling option (kale, collards, chards, spinach, etc.).

Therapeutic herbs: Cooling herbs are particularly beneficial. All warming herbs or heat-retaining herbs should be avoided.

Other healing tonics: Blackberry leaf, chamomile, cat's claw, coriander, chicory, chrysanthemum, comfrey, coriander, calendula, cumin, dandelion root and leaf, fennel, gotu kola, hibiscus, jasmine, lemon, lemon balm, lemon grass, linden, marshmallow, motherwort, nettle, peppermint, raspberry, rose flowers, clover, red root, saffron, skullcap, yellow dock

Limit: Chocolate, salt, meats, nuts, stimulants

Must eliminate: Hot spices, coffee, alcohol, tobacco

Lucky you: Fire bodies can eat delicious sweets! Fire-based constitutions can eat more sweetness than the norm and not be as affected as other types.

AIR/WATER BODY

Energetics: Dry, airy, astringent

Body Components: Lungs, lymph, brain, joints, skin

Chakra: Throat, third eye, crown

Ayurveda: Vata

TCM: Air/Metal

Astrological Rulers: Mercury, Uranus, Neptune

Air/Water body types are ruled by motion. On an annual basis, the most important time for an Air/Water body is in the fall and during the change of seasons. Air/Water is what impels us to change and shift, breaking out of routines into new ones. Those that have a predominance of air and water in their body tend to be very mental, flexible, and creative. These types tend to be very quick and mentally agile, with lots of energy. Air/Water types need to apply routine into their digestive schedule, due to their appetite constantly fluctuating. Their innate craving is for raw and cooling foods, yet because they lack the warming element, this can be detrimental to their joints and muscles, and can also lower their immune systems.

Out of balance, they tend to look depleted, pale, muscle-on-bone thin, fragile, and lanky. Energetically they easily lose willpower, confidence, and boldness. At an older age they naturally enter into a predominantly Air constitution. They start experiencing a drier internal and eternal landscape, wrinkling, and lack of moisture in the limbs, which decreases their mobility and agility.

COMMON CRAVINGS: Raw foods, crunchy, cooling meals

BALANCED CRAVINGS: Warm cooked foods, grounding, sweet and salty flavors

Response to a poor diet: Ungroundedness, fragility, fatigue

Therapeutic foods: The most vital component is establishing a routine with food. Vegetables, particularly root vegetables (beets, carrots, yucca, burdock, sweet potatoes, celeriac, etc.), grains, oats, beans and other legumes, nuts, and seeds are all beneficial. Good fats and oils are a vital component in the Air/Water diet; the most healing oils are good-quality ghee, raw coconut oil, extra virgin olive oil, avocado oil, and flax oil. Steamed dark greens are particularly beneficial. Sweet, ripe, and juicy (nonastringent) fruits are particularly good. Any type of sweetener is okay (except for refined sugar).

Therapeutic herbs: Many herbal teas are good for Air/Water types, yet bitter, astringent, and cooling teas may not be as beneficial. A combination of pungent, grounding, and sweet herbs is best.

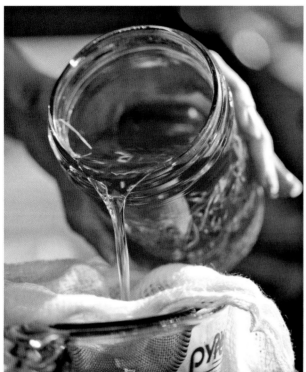 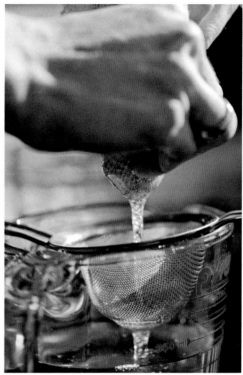

Other healing tonics: Angelica root, bay leaves, cardamom, celery seed and root, cinnamon, cloves, comfrey, elecampane root, fennel root, leaf and seed, gotu kola, fo-ti, ginger, all ginsengs, sarsaparilla, Solomon's seal, wild ginger, yerba santa

Limit: Astringent, stimulating, and cooling foods

Must eliminate: Caffeinated drinks, tobacco, alcohol, excessive raw foods, frozen and canned foods

Lucky you: You get to get away with eating delicious fats and lots of food with such a fast metabolism! Eat lots of good fats and grounding snacks throughout the day to keep your balance.

NEXT-LEVEL CLEANSING

12

Setting Up Your Cleanse

It's always good to begin a cleansing regimen by cleaning the liver. Generally, a body doesn't function optimally whenever a liver is overburdened, yet there is an even greater reason for cleansing the liver first. Until the liver is cleansed, its toxic load will prevent a body from cleansing new toxins and flushing them out. No cleanse will really work unless old liver gunk is cleared out to generate some space. To start cleansing other parts of the body or drinking tonics that assist other organs is partially dysfunctional. If the liver is exhausted, it cannot move cleansing energy to any other part of the body; it is like cleaning a floor with a dirty mop.

The liver and the kidneys maintain a close partnership when cleaning the blood on a regular basis. Toxins are stored inside the liver whenever a body becomes too toxic to excrete them or the materials are too toxic for the kidneys to expel them. In a way, the liver will self-sacrifice when all else fails to defend the rest of the body against antibiotics, heavy metals, chemicals, and other harmful elements. Therefore, many people have extremely impaired livers as a result. The worst toxins are held in the liver and tend to remain there permanently, unless there is an intervention with some heavy-duty practices. A juice cleanse doesn't really do the trick—you certainly need the assistance of tonic herbs, an alkaline diet meal plan, and enemas.

The eventual results of a busy life, a chemical-rich environment, an acid-based diet, and no tonic herbs is a crippled and inflamed liver too impaired to efficiently eliminate future toxins. This is exactly where chronic diseases develop and take over. This is unfortunately very common in the Western world, and this may explain why so many people have major sensitivities to chemicals and allergens. Many believe

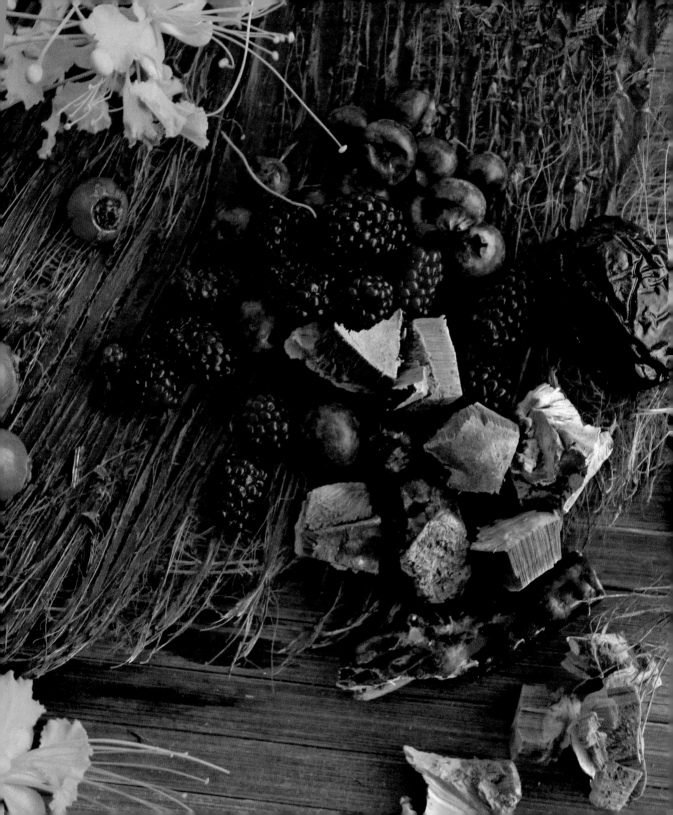

that a major reason for this is heavy chemical treatment of our food, drinking water, and immediate environments. This overburdens the liver with heavy metals that take a long time to flush out. Our livers are resilient machines that can take on quite a lot, so it isn't only because you ate cheeseburger or had a few drinks—it is a combination of eating bad-quality food plus undergoing emotional and environmental stresses.

Many cultures around the world have utilized liquid cleansing, bathing, fasting, and colon cleanses to achieve higher levels of purification for body and mind. Cleanses help us learn to become more intimate with our own body's internal processes. This intimacy goes beyond organs, bones, and joints to our breathing, blood chemistry, vital forces, internal organs, and subtle energies. When we learn to assist our body with its eliminatory processes, we can begin to facilitate the energy of wellness and self-healing.

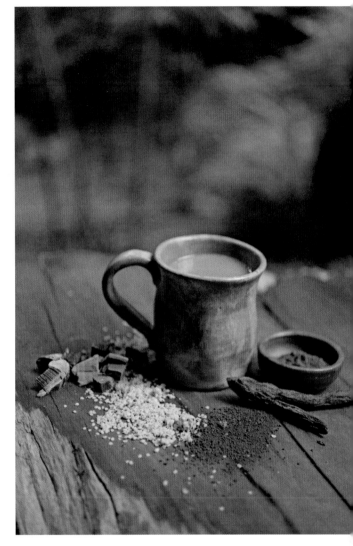

13

Cleansing with Herbal Tonics

Adding tonics to your cleanse routine is easy, yet you must take care when formulating herbs for desired outcomes. Whether you are doing a liquid diet or a particular dietary routine, add two or three tonics within your day to keep you fueled. Keep in mind not to overdo many herbs—the more you concentrate on a set of herbs, the more you should track the effects within yourself, as well as thoroughly cleansing the organs you are targeting.

Add up to four of these herbs to your cleanse schedule, from one or two categories, and use juices that go well with the category you are choosing. In the recipe section, each juice cocktail is delineated with the category in which it fits. This way you can custom-make your cleanse to fit your needs.

FORMULAS FOR CLEANSING HEALTH

Make these formulas to add to your own cleanse to boost this particular area in your body. If you are looking to detox and mineralize your liver, follow the suggested liver herbs, or if you are seeking to shed a few pounds, add the weight-loss herbs into your cleansing regime.

Herbs for skin and hair: Horsetail, gotu kola, calendula, fo-ti, turmeric

Herbs for weight loss: Garcinia cambogia, green coffee bean, cha de bugre, turmeric, mangosteen, hibiscus, schisandra berries

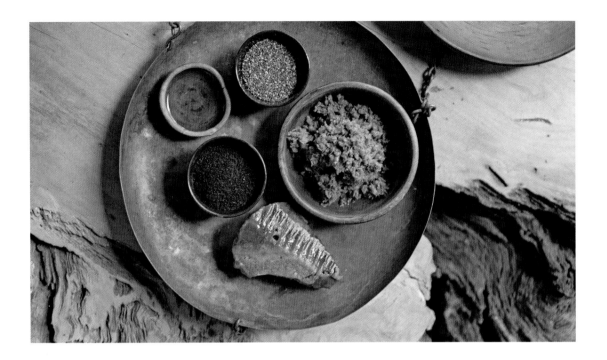

Herbs for liver and gall bladder:
Artichoke leaf, chanca piedra, milk thistle seed, dandelion root and leaf, burdock root, turmeric root, nettle leaf and seed, fennel root, Oregon grape root, yellow dock, quassia bark, rue, lemon peel, spirulina

Herbs for the stomach and colon:
Slippery elm, chia, gynostemma, tulsi, marshmallow root, cat's claw

Herbs for kidneys: Horsetail, marshmallow root, chanca piedra, parsley seed and leaf, schisandra berries, gynostemma, dandelion

Herbs for anti-stress: Rhodiola, all medicinal mushrooms (reishi, chaga, shiitake, maiitake, etc.), gynostemma, schisandra berries, ginseng

Herbs for candida: Pau d'arco, reishi, chaga, sangre de drago, jergón sacha

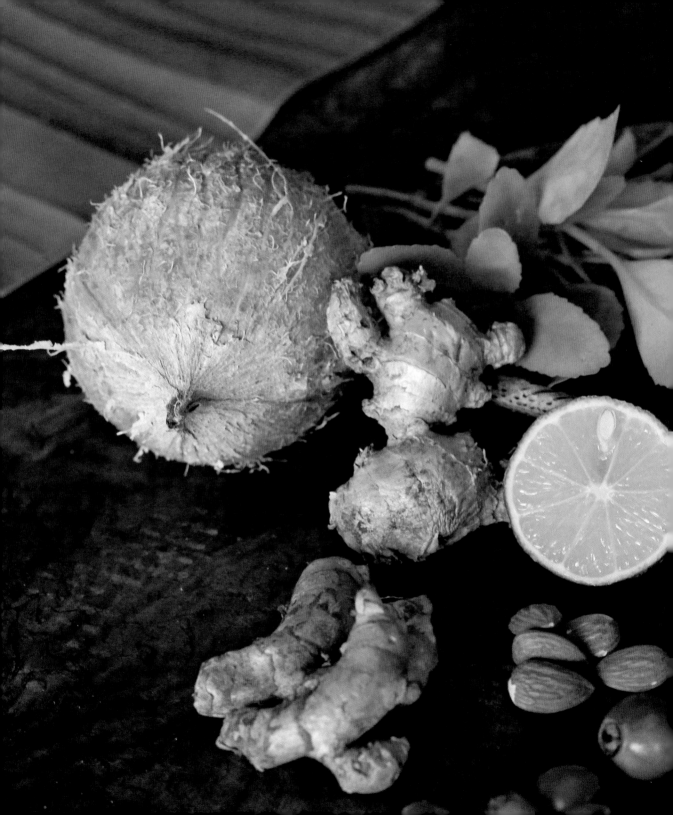

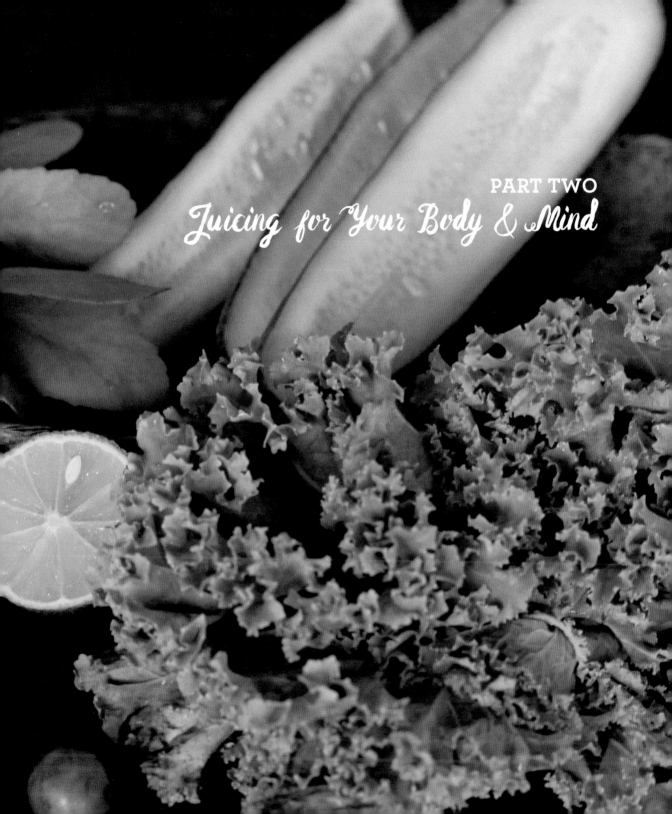

PART TWO

Juicing for Your Body & Mind

JUICE RECIPES

Before we start our healing juice journey, there are a few things to keep in mind. The recipes are broken down into two main sections. Part 1 will show how to prepare a basic juice combination as well as what type of preparation it can be. Part 2, "Juice Sensorium," will be a more strictly medicinal section that will target specific healing qualities.

Be sure to keep the following basics in mind when preparing your healing juices.

BUYING ORGANIC PRODUCE & HERBS

It is smart to invest in this for yourself, because not only do you deserve it, but this is truly your healthcare. If you really want to see the positive effects of good food on your health, then treat the fruit, vegetables, and herbs you buy as your medicine. I promise that you'll feel the vibrational and physical difference by choosing this lifestyle. If your budget doesn't always permit it, then be wise when choosing your staple fruits and veggies. You can abide by the "dirty dozen" suggestions for avoiding the worst nonorganic foods: apples, strawberries, grapes, celery, spinach, cucumbers, red bell peppers, nectarines, peaches, tomatoes, blueberries, and potatoes. But if you can manage it, of course you should try to have all your daily favorites be organic. Usually a lower-cost and higher-quality alternative is to buy your produce at the local farmers market.

STICKING TO FRESHNESS

Have your juice daily. If you can, always prepare your own juice and drink it immediately or shortly after preparation. The nutritional content of the juice within the first minutes after it has been made is powerfully loaded with oxygen, phytonutrients, and sensitive enzymatic catalyzers. Cold-pressed juice naturally preserves better than other methods of preparation and is good for about 2 days. If you are using a centrifugal juicer, don't allow more than an hour or so to go by before consumption. Because centrifugal juicers generate heat, the juice doesn't have as much fiber per liquid ounce as a cold-pressed juice; also because of oxidization the molecular integrity is lost much more quickly.

DRINKING YOUR TONICS DAILY

I believe that juice is much more effective in delivering healing properties when it is consumed on a regular basis. It is important to keep a solid routine with your juice, and I believe in rotating your medicines to correspond to the issues you may be facing in body and mind.

As a general rule of thumb, make your tonics with higher amounts of veggies than fruit. Fruit juice is a fantastic source of energy and essential sugars, but still be sure to incorporate high quantities of leafy greens and other veggies in your diet. If you keep your veggies at a higher percentage of your daily diet and use low-glycemic fruits, you'll feel the difference.

EATING WITH THE SEASONS

The body's functions are perfectly synchronized with seasonal rhythms, meaning we can benefit most from fruits and vegetables that are at their peak at any given time. Don't worry about not having readily available ingredients that are called for within some recipes. Other fruits or veggies can be substituted. Be flexible with your bioavailability, and listen to the intuitive aspects of what your body wants and needs. Of course, having worldwide availability of superfoods, tonic herbs, and fruits is alluring, yet first things first: use what you have. Don't stress, and take the time to discover new superherbs that grow in your area.

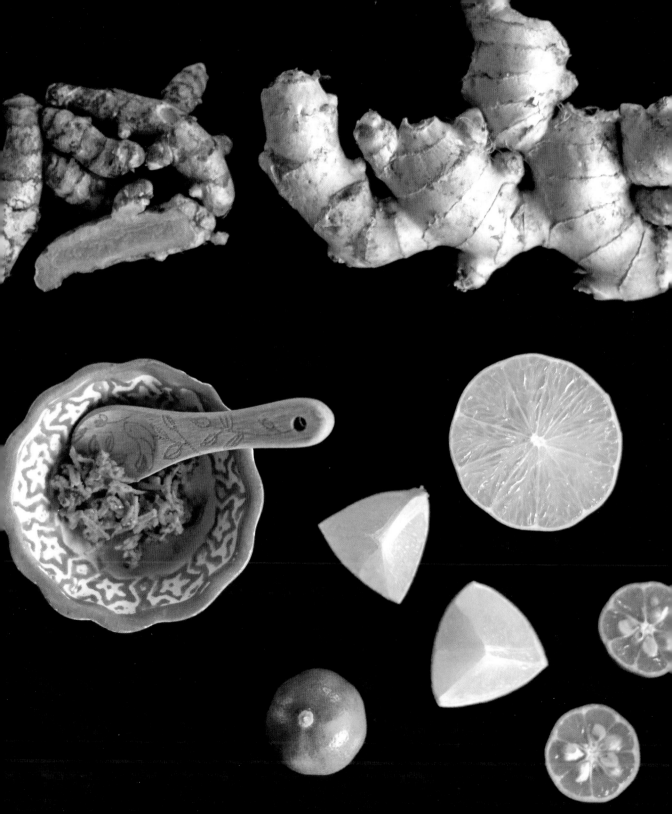

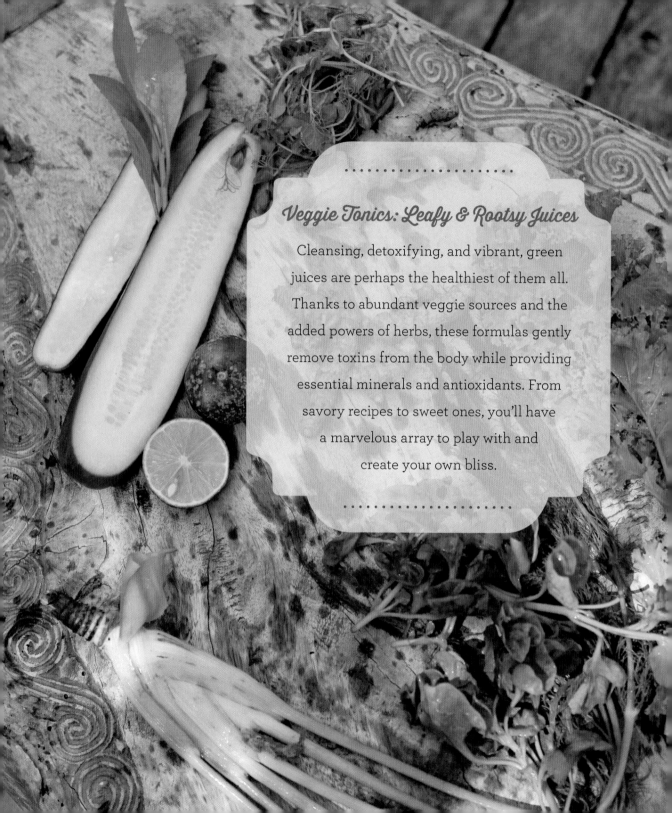

Veggie Tonics: Leafy & Rootsy Juices

Cleansing, detoxifying, and vibrant, green juices are perhaps the healthiest of them all. Thanks to abundant veggie sources and the added powers of herbs, these formulas gently remove toxins from the body while providing essential minerals and antioxidants. From savory recipes to sweet ones, you'll have a marvelous array to play with and create your own bliss.

EASIEST GREEN JUICE

This is a great base recipe to work from. This is the best kind of simple juice, made with ingredients that you should always have on hand. Use this recipe as a basis from which to work. This is a great start-off green juice that will get your green needs fulfilled. One serving provides the essential alkalinity, antioxidants, and mineralization needed in a meal.

Makes 1 serving

> 6 ounces pineapple
> 4 ounces celery
> 4 ounces kale
> ½ ounce lemon
> 1 ounce ginger
>
> **Optional:** Add 1 ounce dandelion greens and a pinch of cayenne to boost its blood-building power.

1. Add all ingredients to your juicer, and blend.

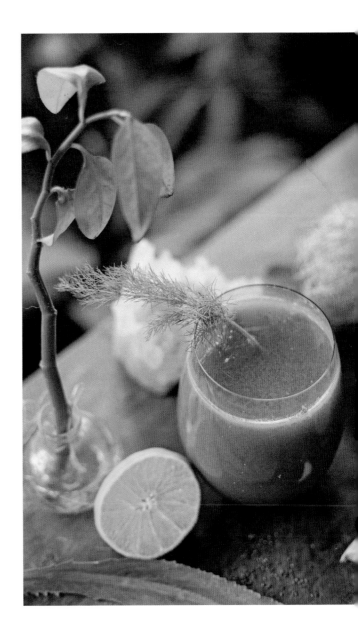

MASTER ALKALIZER

Our body's internal system needs a pH just above 7.0. We call this range alkaline. Our enzymatic, immunologic, and repair mechanisms all function their best in this alkaline range. However, our metabolic processes—the processes of living, tissue repair, and the metabolism of food—produce a great deal of acid. In order to maintain our internal alkaline state, we need our daily greens and herbal tonics to stay alkaline and curb cravings!

Makes 1 serving

1 cup kale
1 cup spinach
2 stalks celery
1 cucumber
Handful dandelion leaf
Handful parsley
1 small burdock root
1 teaspoon turmeric root

1. Add all ingredients to your juicer, and blend.

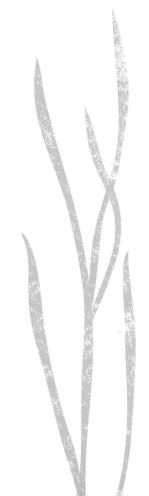

GALL BLADDER FLUSH

This is another recipe that can be used to flush out a body organ—in this case, the gall bladder.

   1 coconut
   1 teaspoon aloe water
   ½ ounce lemon juice
   1 teaspoon turmeric powder
   1 teaspoon chanca piedra powder*

1. Crack open a fresh coconut and extract the coconut water. Place 6 ounces of the coconut water in a glass.

2. Add the remaining ingredients to the blender, blend and then pour into glass.

---

* The Spanish name of the plant *chanca piedra* means "stone breaker" or "shatter stone." It was named for its effective use to generations of Amazonian and Central American indigenous peoples in eliminating gallstones and kidney stones.

GROUNDING CLEANSER

While cleansing, sometimes we feel like we are losing it. We feel out of it, headachy, and a bit anxious or fatigued, and we need a little extra something to tide us over without losing the cleanse's focus. This drink will keep the side effects of the cleanse at bay while providing clarity and strength so you can continue to access its benefits.

Makes 1 serving

   1 coconut
   ½ avocado
   ½ cup sprouted cashews
   1 cup fresh kale
   1 cups pineapple
   1 teaspoon graviola powder
   1 teaspoon chanca piedra powder
   1 teaspoon spirulina powder

1. Crack open a fresh coconut and extract the coconut water. Place 8 ounces of the coconut water in a glass.

2. Add the remaining ingredients to the juicer, and blend.

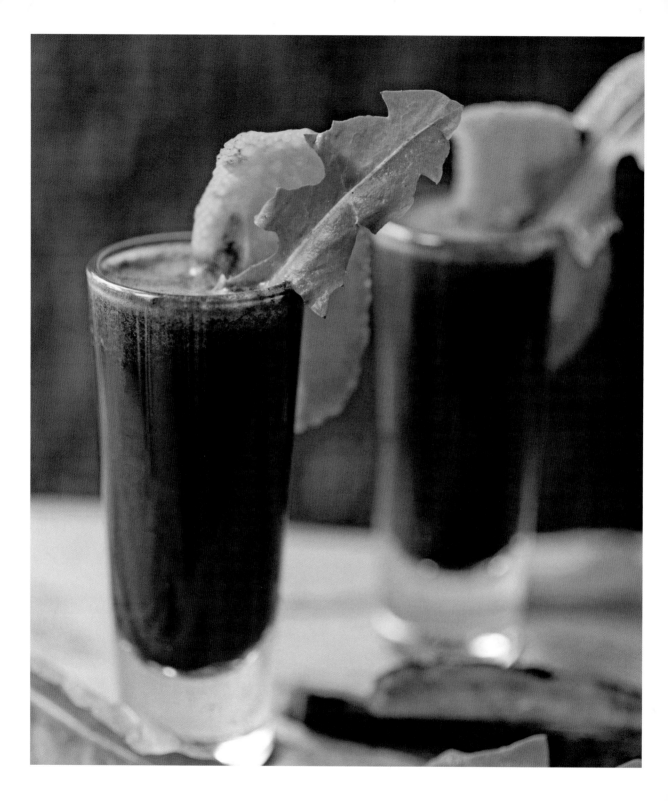

DR. RAINFOREST

This is a bold and deeply mineralizing juice. This juice is inspired by rainforest traditions that incorporate moringa and graviola into the daily cleansing. These two rainforest staples have a long, rich history of use in herbal medicine as well as a lengthy recorded indigenous use. From the Peruvian Andes to Costa Rica, they both have been used traditionally for liver problems and stomach imbalances. Externally it has also been traditionally applied as a bandage as well as to help treat neuralgia, rheumatism, and arthritis pain.

Makes 1 serving

   1 aloe leaf
   2 ounces water
   4 ounces dandelion leaf
   Handful parsley
   Handful cilantro
   4 ounces kale
   1 ounce lemon
   1 teaspoon moringa powder
   1 teaspoon graviola powder

1. Make fresh aloe water: scrape about 1–2 teaspoons of goo from inside of the aloe leaf. Blend with 2 ounces of water.

2. Juice the dandelion leaf, parsley, cilantro, kale, and lemon.

3. Add the moringa and graviola, and mix all ingredients together. Add to a juicer, and blend.

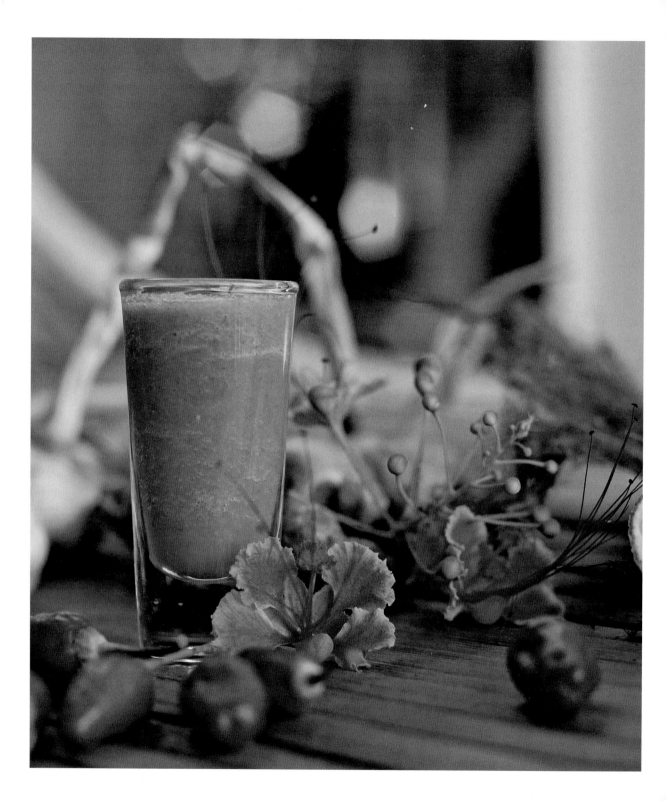

FLU SHOT

This shot will kick your system into shape. I call this the "antivenom" shot; it'll help you fight the roughest colds, throat infections, and any annoying virus that may have caught you.

Makes 1 shot

1 teaspoon cold-pressed garlic juice
2 teaspoons ginger, finely grated
1 teaspoon fresh squeezed lemon juice
1 teaspoon apple cider vinegar
¼ teaspoon pau d'arco powder
1 ounce aloe water (ideally, fresh)
Pinch cayenne
Pinch pink salt

Optional: 10 drops of dragon blood (*sangre de drago*) extract.

Note: *Sangre de grado's* red sap has a long history of indigenous use across the rainforests of Latin America. In the early 1600s, Spanish naturalist Padre Bernabé Cobo found that the curative power of the sap was widely known throughout the indigenous tribes of Mexico, Costa Rica, Peru, and Ecuador. For centuries, the sap has been painted on wounds to staunch bleeding, to accelerate healing, and to seal and protect injuries from infection. The sap dries quickly and forms a barrier, much like a "second skin."

1. Mix all ingredients, together. Add to a juicer, and blend.

KIDNEY FLUSH

This is a refreshing and gentle approach to a morning kidney flush.

Makes 1 serving

1 coconut
1 teaspoon aloe water
½ ounce lemon juice
1 teaspoon solé

1. Crack open a fresh coconut and extract the coconut water. Place 6 ounces of the coconut water in a glass.

2. Add the remaining ingredients to the blender, blend, and enjoy.

Solé

In a mason jar, add 6 large pink salt crystals, and fill with water. This is a great way to take your salt; have it on your countertop any time you need it for your herbal drinks. The salt will eventually dissolve and infuse into the water. It is an excellent tonic to nourish the kidneys. Recommended dosage is 1 teaspoon added to your water or juice.

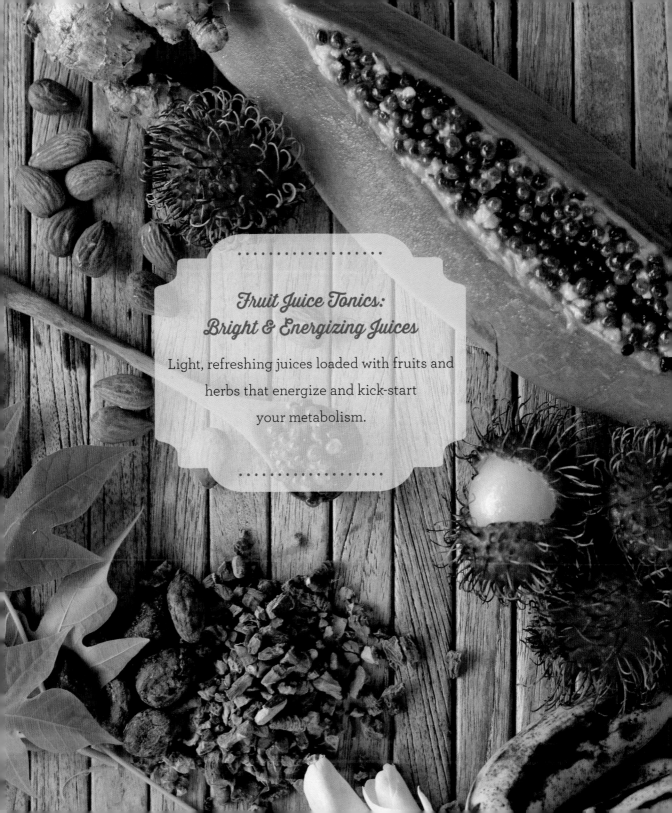

Fruit Juice Tonics:
Bright & Energizing Juices

Light, refreshing juices loaded with fruits and
herbs that energize and kick-start
your metabolism.

PIÑA COLADA WITH A TWIST

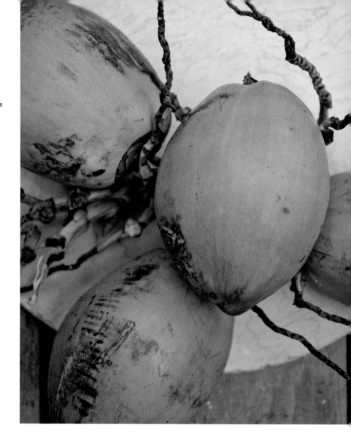

The traditional Piña Colada recipe was originally created to be a gentle liver-boosting recipe. Pineapple is used to decrease inflammation, and coconut to nourish and mineralize. Without the booze, piña coladas are actually an amazing liver tonic—a liver detox/retox cocktail that won't kill you with a terrible hangover! In this recipe I add cilantro to assist the liver in heavy-metal removal, and some orange peel to soothe the gut.

Makes 2 servings

1 whole pineapple
1 coconut
1 cup cilantro leaves
Orange peel shavings
Honey or agave (optional)

1. Cold-press the pineapple, collecting about 8 ounces of juice.

2. Crack open the coconut, and drain the liquid into a blender. Then scrape about 1 cup of coconut meat out. Blend the coconut meat and coconut water until it reaches a creamy consistency. Remove all but ½ cup of this mixture from the blender, and reserve it for another use.

3. Add the cilantro (less if you'd like a little less predominant flavor), orange peel, and honey to the blender, and blend until smooth.

BERRIES 'N' PEELS

Within these berries and peels you will find an astonishingly powerful source of vitamin C. Camu camu, mangosteen, and açai are the rainforest's most treasured fruits; they contain a megaload of antioxidants, phytochemicals, and minerals.

Makes 1–2 servings

1 cup frozen blueberries
1 cup frozen açai
1 frozen banana
1 teaspoon mangosteen peel powder
1 teaspoon camu camu peel powder
2 cups water
1–2 dates

1. Blend all ingredients together, and enjoy!

Note: Camu camu is the one of most loved fruits of the rainforest, and it has the highest recorded amount of natural vitamin C known on the planet. In comparison to an orange, a camu camu provides thirty times more vitamin C, ten times more iron, three times more niacin, twice as much riboflavin, and half again as much more phosphorus.

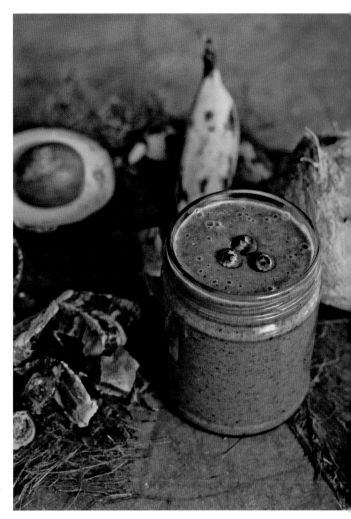

ENERGY ELIXIR

I love combining blood sugar regulators with fruits. Pau d'arco and cat's claw are rainforest master tonics commonly used throughout the rainforest for their anticandidal and antimicrobial properties. In addition to having many other abilities, it will regulate your blood sugar and curb sweet cravings in general. Having a fruit smoothie with this herbal assistance is the best way to metabolize sugar and put your hormones in balance. Many tribes in Costa Rica, Peru, and Brazil, have called it the "divine tree." According to the herbalist Leslie Taylor, "It helps to increase red blood cell production and helps respiratory disorders, ulcers, candida excess, and athlete's foot."

Note: Throughout Central and South America, many different tribes have employed pau d'arco, using it for the same purposes for generations.

Makes 1–2 servings

1½ cups almond milk (see below)
1 large frozen banana
1 cup frozen blueberries
2 tablespoons hemp seeds
2 tablespoons cacao nibs
1 cup kale, tightly packed
1 teaspoon cat's claw powder
1 teaspoon pau d'arco powder

1. Blend all ingredients together, and enjoy!

Nut Milk

Nut milk is used in a number of recipes in this book. It's easy to make your own. Ideally, soak the nuts in water for 1–2 hours before making the milk. In a blender, combine ½ cup nuts with 2 cups water. Strain the milk with cheesecloth, and press the pulp. If you opt to use store-bought nut milk, be sure to choose one that is unsweetened.

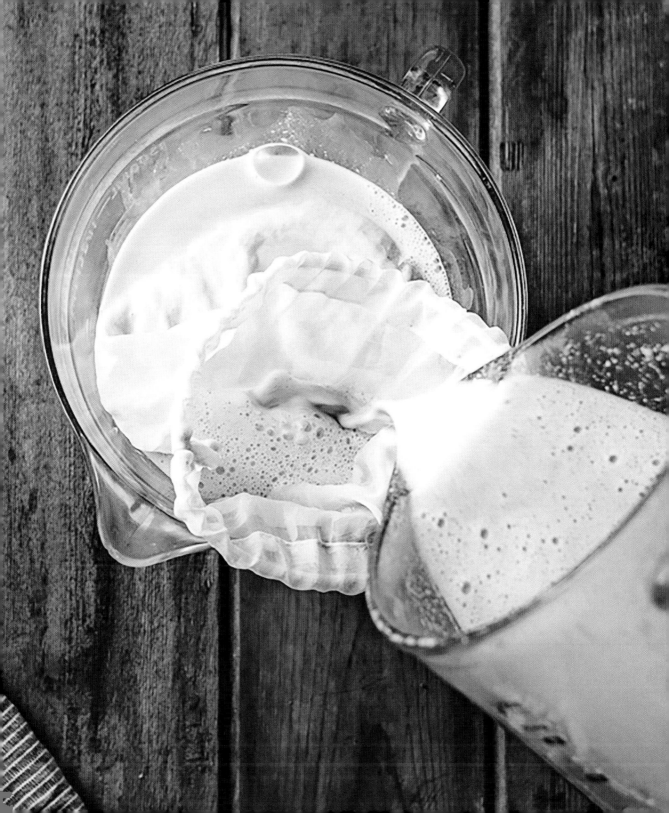

ENERGIZING BEET TONIC

1 beet
1 cucumber
2 green apples
1 ginger knob
1 teaspoon ginseng extract

1. Juice the beet, cucumber, apples, and ginger. Combine the juices in a shaker.

2. Add the ginseng extract and shake well.

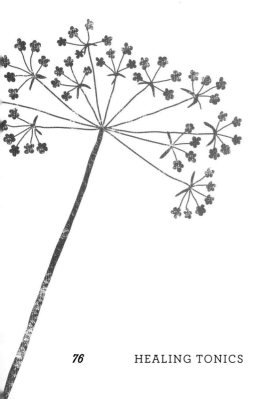

WOMEN'S TONIC

This fruity and bright tonic is meant to balance the hormonal fluctuations of the moon. The black cohosh and wild yam are powerful herbs from the North and South that studies have shown support a healthy uterus. Many treat fertility as if it were something to fear or inherently negative, unless you want to get pregnant. Well, the fact is that fertile means "healthy." It's like picking a juicy fruit, perfectly ripe and colorful, loaded with seeds, and then denying it. We want our fruit to have seeds and be a vibrant source of nutrients. In native rainforest cultures, fertility is a sign of being truly healthy and in balance with nature. To most rainforest tribal peoples, fertility determines a balanced heart and mind. This recipe is drawn upon a classic Central American native formula for men and women to enhance the body with essential fertility.

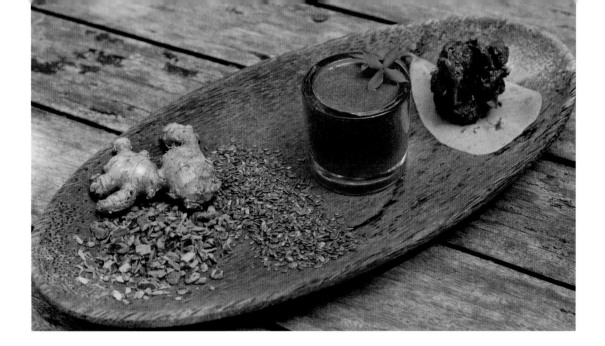

Makes 2–3 servings

12 ounces cold-pressed watermelon juice
6 ounces fresh coconut water
4 ounces beet root juice
2 ounces ginger juice
3 fresh rose hips, juiced (or ½ teaspoon
  dried powder)
½ teaspoon black cohosh extract (or
  1 teaspoon dried powder)
1 teaspoon wild yam extract (or
  1 teaspoon dried powder)
½ teaspoon muira puama powder
Ice

1. Combine the watermelon juice, coconut water, beet root juice, ginger juice, and rose hip juice. Stir.

2. Combine the liquid mixture with the rest of the ingredients: black cohosh, wild yam, and muira puama. If you are using rose hip powder rather than fresh rose hips, add it at this point.

3. Pour into a shaker over ice, shake, strain into glasses, and enjoy.

Note: Muira puama is also called "potency wood." In Brazilian herbal medicine, muira puama still is a highly regarded sexual stimulant with a reputation as a powerful aphrodisiac. It is used as a neuromuscular tonic for sexual weakness and menstrual disturbances, sexual impotency, and central nervous system disorders.

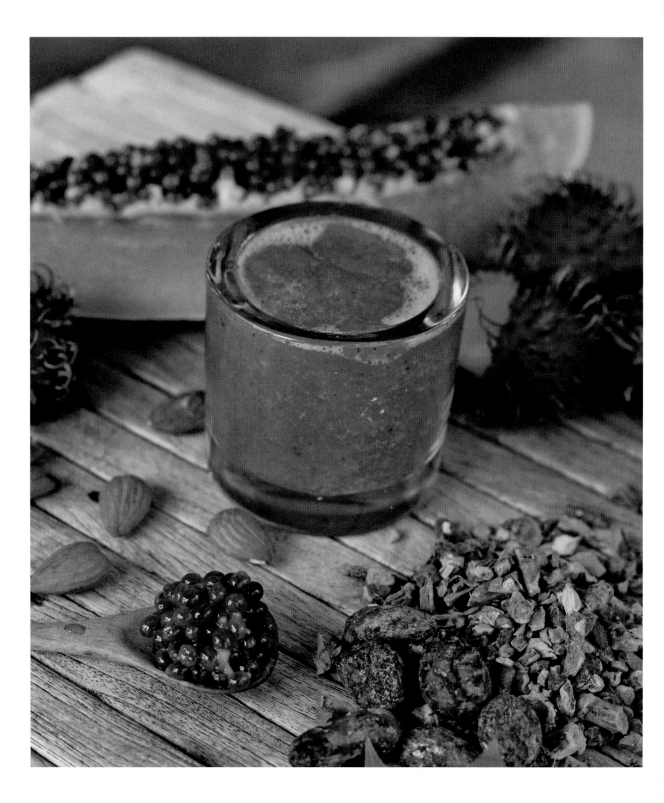

MEN'S TONIC

It is of vital importance for men to keep their prostate healthy and fertile. Most men as they age encounter some sort of prostate condition. This walnut-size gland sitting right below the bladder is in charge of providing nourishment to the semen, overall circulation to the muscles, and elimination (ejaculation). To keep a strong virility, men need to care for their seeds and make sure they keep a fertile makeup in order to prevent any issues when aging. Saw palmetto, suma, and yohimbe are master tonics known to enhance vigor, energize, and boost potency to the prostate.

Makes 2 servings

1 cup almond milk (see page 74)
1 cup chopped papaya
1 teaspoon fresh papaya seeds
4 rambutans,* peeled
1 tablespoon cacao nibs
1 teaspoon muira puama powder
1 teaspoon suma root powder
½ teaspoon yohimbe powder
1 date

1. Blend all ingredients together, and enjoy!

Note: In South America suma is known as *para toda* (which means "for all things") and as Brazilian ginseng. Suma root has been used for generations as an adaptogen and regenerative tonic. It is also a master energizer to treat exhaustion, chornic fatigue, libido, diabetes, and cancer recovery, and as a general cure-all for many types of illnesses.

---

* If you cannot find rambutans, substitute 1 cup frozen blueberries.

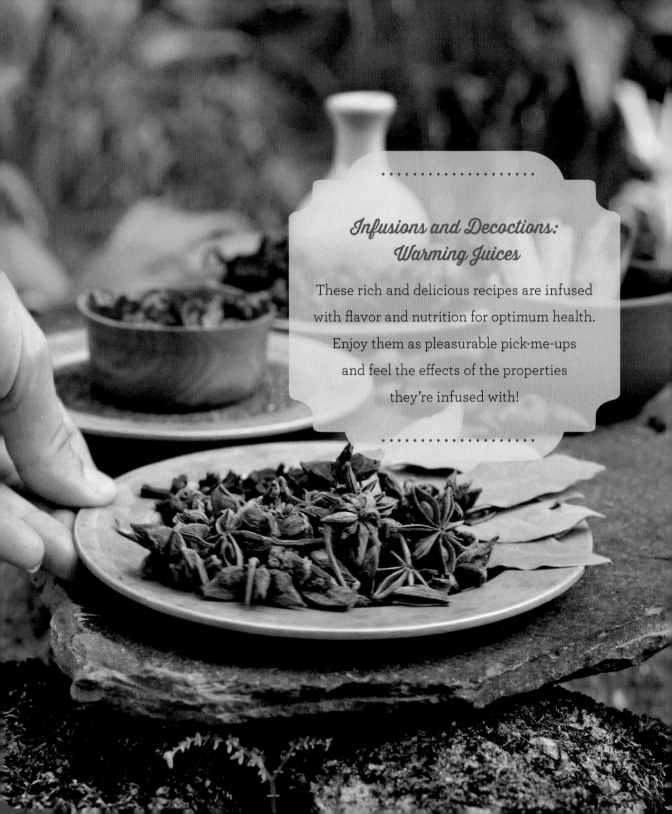

Infusions and Decoctions: Warming Juices

These rich and delicious recipes are infused
with flavor and nutrition for optimum health.
Enjoy them as pleasurable pick-me-ups
and feel the effects of the properties
they're infused with!

REISHI HOT CHOCOLATE

This sweet and spicy mug of cocoa also has the immune-enhancing power of reishi.

Note: Reishi mushroom is used for boosting the immune system, from *viral infections* to *lung* conditions including *asthma* and *bronchitis;* It has also greatly contributed to reducing *heart disease* and contributing conditions such as *high blood pressure* and *high cholesterol.*

Makes 1 serving

>   1 teaspoon reishi mushroom powder
>   2–3 tablespoons cacao powder
>   1 teaspoon coconut oil
>   ¼ teaspoon cinnamon
>   1 teaspoon vanilla
>   1 pinch of cayenne
>   Hot water
>   Milk of choice

1. Mix the reishi, cacao, coconut oil, cinnamon, vanilla, and cayenne into a cup of hot water, and mix well. Add your milk of choice.

CHAGA CHAI

This spicy and warming chai has potent healing power. Chai has been considered an aromatic master nourisher for centuries, known for its ability to prepare the stomach for digestion. It is commonly consumed before and after meals to flush the system with healing spices.

Makes 1 serving

4 cups water
½ teaspoon cinnamon
1 knob fresh ginger
A few cloves
1 teaspoon chaga
1 teaspoon roasted dandelion root
1 teaspoon Earl Grey black tea (omit for a caffeine-free beverage)
1 teaspoon cardamom pods
1 teaspoon vanilla powder (or extract)
½ cup choice of nut milk

Note: Chaga is now being extensively studied as one of the most effective sources to prevent tumor growth.

1. Place the water in a pot, and bring the cinnamon, ginger, cloves, chaga, and roasted dandelion root to a boil.

2. After about 15 minutes, lower the heat and add the tea, cardamom, and vanilla. Allow it to infuse for about 10 minutes, and strain.

3. Add your choice of nut milk and sweetener.

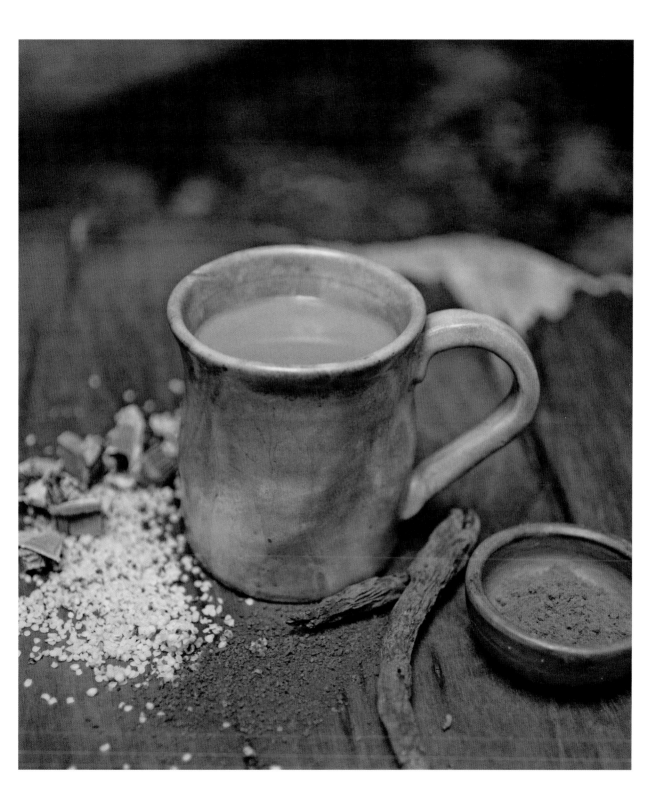

FLOWER VITAMIN WATER

The pharmacy of flowers contains a variety of healing properties. The tradition of flower essences is as old as the history of medicine. Did you know that adding herbs and flowers to your water naturally filters and enhances the electrolyte power of your water? This simple act not only beautifies one of the most special resources of the body but also provides the best form of hydration.

Note: In Costa Rican native traditions, flower waters were used for energetic *limpias*, also known as spirit cleanses. Traditionally medicine women would prepare the flower water to bathe somone to cleanse them from bad energy, evil eye, and emotional imbalance. The treatment is considered to be a form of spiritual rebirth that is meant to be done on a regular basis.

Makes 2–3 servings

> 2 quarts filtered water
> 2–3 sprigs fresh chamomile flowers
> 1 sprig fresh rosemary
> 2–3 sprigs fresh lavender

1. Fill a large glass vessel or bottle with the filtered water.

2. Add the whole herbs, with stems, into the water.

3. Place in the fridge to chill, or add ice before drinking.

MUSCLE AND JOINT TONIC

This grounding herbal tea tonic contains horsetail and comfrey, potent tonics
known to support bone strength, tissue recovery, and toning.

Makes 1 serving

> 2 cups water
> 1 ounce lemon juice
> 4 ounces comfrey leaf
> 4 ounces horsetail leaf

1. In a pot, bring the water to a boil.

2. Add the lemon juice, comfrey, and horsetail. Simmer for 20–30 minutes.

3. Strain and enjoy!

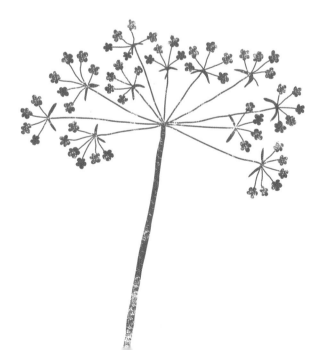

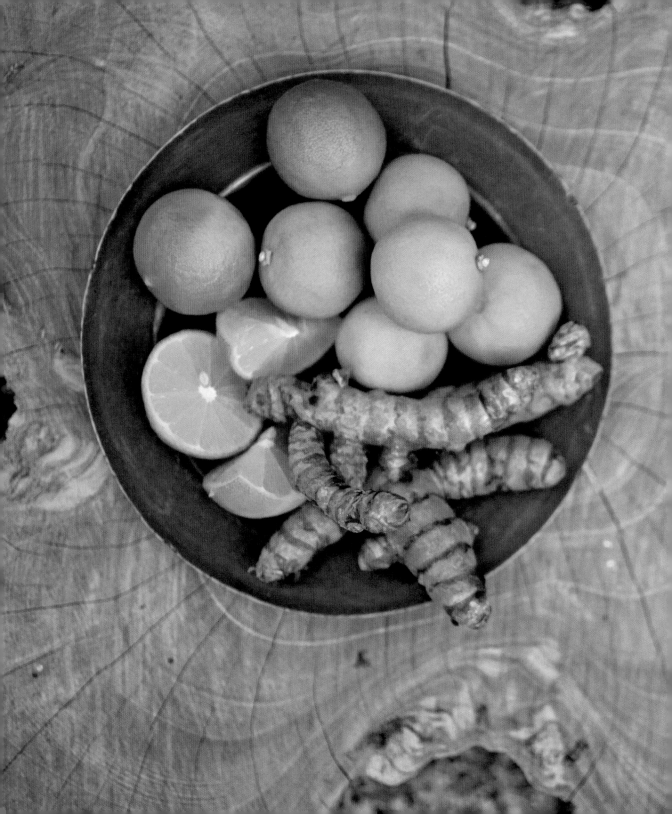

TURMERIC DETOX WATER

This detox water is a hydrating and anti-inflammatory drink to have throughout the day.

Makes 1–2 servings

1 teaspoon turmeric
1 ounce lemon juice
12 ounces water
1 ounce cold-pressed ginger
1 teaspoon honey or maple syrup
Ice (optional)

1. Add the turmeric and lemon juice to the water, and stir well.

2. Add the ginger and honey, and mix well.

3. Add ice cubes or place in the fridge to chill. This formula can also be made with warm water instead of ice. Enjoy!

PISTACHIO MESQUITE MILK

This is an exquisite, energizing, and healing milk with the grounding touch of mesquite and ashwagandha for strength and stamina.

2½ cups pistachio milk (see page 74)
1 tablespoon mesquite powder
1 tablespoon ashwagandha powder
1 tablespoon honey or other sweetener

1. Blend all ingredients, and enjoy!

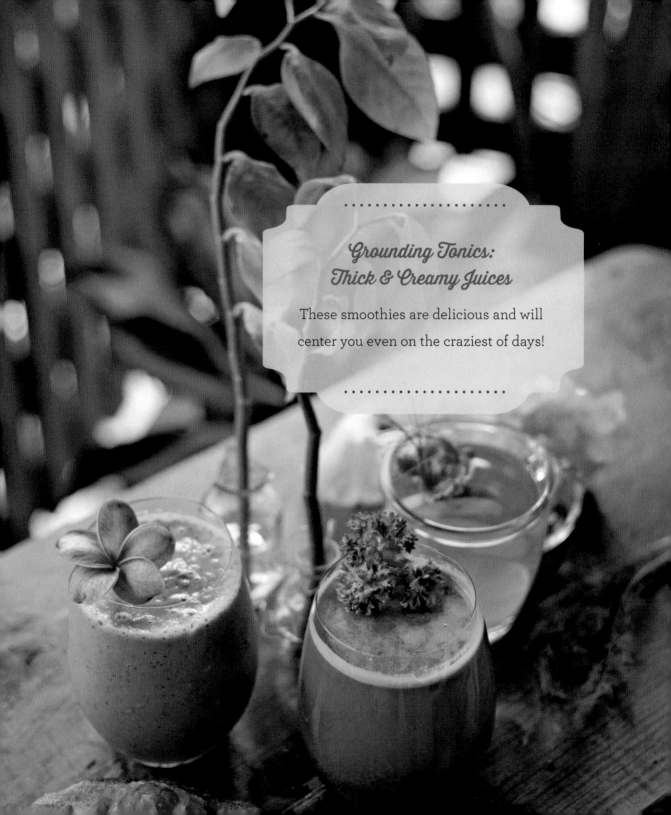

Grounding Tonics:
Thick & Creamy Juices

These smoothies are delicious and will center you even on the craziest of days!

MUSHROOM CHOCOLATE SMOOTHIE

Ahhh ... one of my absolute favorites. This is one of those exquisite tonic smoothies that can be consumed daily. It's hard to get tired of this one, and your body will always be able to take advantage of the nutrients it provides. This smoothie contains immense immune-boosting power, necessary minerals for the day, and enough dopamine to boost you with mental energy. Mushrooms make miracle tonics that facilitate a total body healing experience.

Makes 1–2 servings

3 frozen bananas (peel before putting them in the freezer)
2 dates
1 tablespoon honey or coconut sugar
2 tablespoons cacao powder
1 teaspoon reishi powder
1 teaspoon chaga
½ teaspoon mangosteen peel
2 cups almond milk (see page 74)
⅓ teaspoon cinnamon
Pinch cayenne
Handful ice cubes

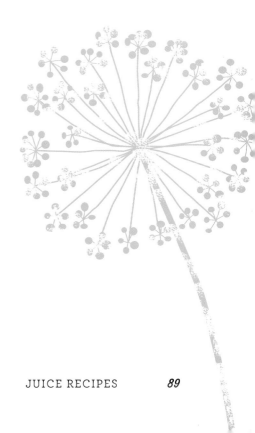

1. Blend all ingredients until smooth.

GOLDEN MILK

You'll enjoy this creamy anti-inflammatory milk, which has a nourishing touch of turmeric.

Makes 2–3 servings

> 2 cups cashew milk (see page 74)
> 1 tablespoon turmeric powder
> 1 pinch of black pepper
> ½ teaspoon cinnamon
> 1 date
> Stevia or maple syrup to taste (optional)

Note: Adding black pepper optimizes the absorption of turmeric, enhancing its medicinal potential within the body.

1. In a blender, combine the cashew milk, turmeric, pepper, cinnamon, and date. Blend well.

2. Taste, and add stevia if needed to reach your desired level of sweetness.

LIVER CLEANSER

Makes 1 serving

> 1 cup pineapple chunks
> 1 whole passion fruit
> ½ avocado
> ½ cup parsley
> 1 cup kale
> 1 teaspoon lemon juice
> 1 teaspoon moringa powder
> 1 teaspoon graviola powder
> ½ cup ice
> Water, as needed

1. Blend all ingredients until smooth, adjusting the amount of water to reach the desired consistency.

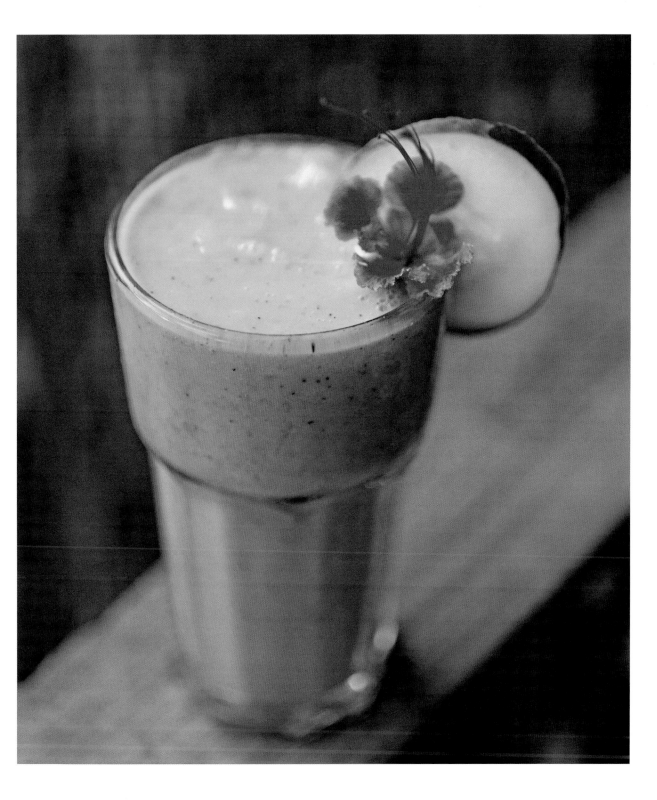

GOJI AND MORINGA SMOOTHIE

This energizing and highly mineralizing smoothie combines the sweetness of green grapes and goji berries. Costa Rican indigenous peoples drink green coffee bean tea to enhance their energy and strength. A tea is commonly taken in the morning before they cross long and difficult distances over the mountains.

Note: Green coffee beans have a higher level of chlorogenic acid compared to regular roasted coffee beans. Chlorogenic acid in green coffee is thought to have health benefits for *heart disease*, diabetes, *weight loss*, among other things.

Makes 1 serving

   1 cup kale
   2 frozen bananas
   ¼ cup dried goji berries
   2 cups frozen green grapes
   1 teaspoon moringa powder
   1 teaspoon green coffee beans
   1–2 cups water

1. Blend ingredients until smooth.

SUPER IRON SMOOTHIE

This energizing smoothie is also rich in iron.

Makes 1 serving

   Handful dinosaur (lacinato) kale (or other dark leafy green)
   Handful spinach
   1 celery stick
   ½ medium-sized cucumber
   1 handful herbs (parsley, cilantro, dandelion leaf)
   1 knob ginger, chopped
   1 teaspoon nourishing mother tonic (see recipe on page 131)
   1 teaspoon spirulina
   1 teaspoon chlorella
   Pinch salt
   Juice of ½ lemon or lime
   1 cup fresh coconut water or water
   2–3 dates, or a bit of agave
   1 frozen banana, chopped

1. Blend all ingredients together until creamy and smooth, and enjoy!

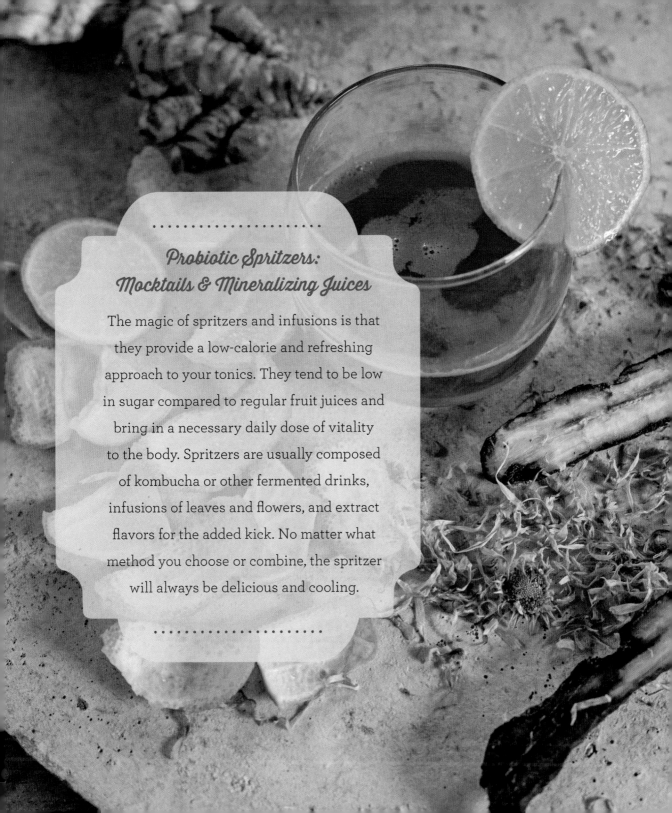

Probiotic Spritzers:
Mocktails & Mineralizing Juices

The magic of spritzers and infusions is that they provide a low-calorie and refreshing approach to your tonics. They tend to be low in sugar compared to regular fruit juices and bring in a necessary daily dose of vitality to the body. Spritzers are usually composed of kombucha or other fermented drinks, infusions of leaves and flowers, and extract flavors for the added kick. No matter what method you choose or combine, the spritzer will always be delicious and cooling.

SCHISANDRA GINGER PROBIOTIC SPRITZ

This refreshing and tart tonic with a spicy punch contains a healthy serving of probiotics to restore alkalinity and boost gut health.

Makes 2 servings

> 2 cups water
> ½ cup schisandra berries
> 8 ounces regular kombucha* (unflavored)
> 4 ounces cold-pressed ginger
> 2 teaspoons lemon juice
> 8 ounces sparkling water
> Agave or stevia

1. Bring the water to a boil. Add the schisandra berries to the pot, and simmer for about 30 minutes. Once about ½–1 cup of the water has evaporated, filter.

2. Mix the ginger juice, lemon juice, and kombucha into the berry infusion, then divide between two glasses.

3. Divide the sparking water between the two glasses, and sweeten with agave to taste.

* Choose any regular unflavored kombucha you like.

GYNOSTEMMA BASIL SPARKLING LEMONADE

Gynostemma is a quintessential tonic, known as the "miracle green" leaf. This is one of Asia's premier longevity herbs, treasured for its anti-aging and antioxidant properties. Among gynastemma's miraculous properties is support of healthy activity in the immune system. Traditionally it has been revered for its cardiovascular and digestive effects. Many love this tonic for its ability to immediately soothe the gut, which makes it a great post-digestive tea. Its naturally sweet flavor makes it a great herb to essentially use for just about anything.

Makes 2 servings

2 tablespoons gynostemma
2 cups almost boiling water
2 ounces lemon juice
Maple syrup, stevia, or other
   sweetener
Ice
Handful fresh basil
8 ounces sparkling water

Note: Gynsotemma, also known as jiaogulan, is an adaptogen and antioxidant whose chemical constituents (saponins) have similar properties to ginseng. The tea is valued for its antioxidant protection and cardiovascular benefits.

1. Add the gynostemma to the water. Allow it to steep for about 15 minutes, then strain.

2. Put the tea in the fridge to cool, or wait until it's lukewarm.

3. Add the lemon juice.

4. Sweeten with maple syrup to taste.

5. Fill glasses with ice cubes and basil leaves, pour in your mix, and top with sparkling water.

Note: The more these types of mixtures sit in the fridge, the better they get. If you make a larg batch and add everything except the ice, within 24 hours the basil infuses its exquisite subtle taste into the gynostemma.

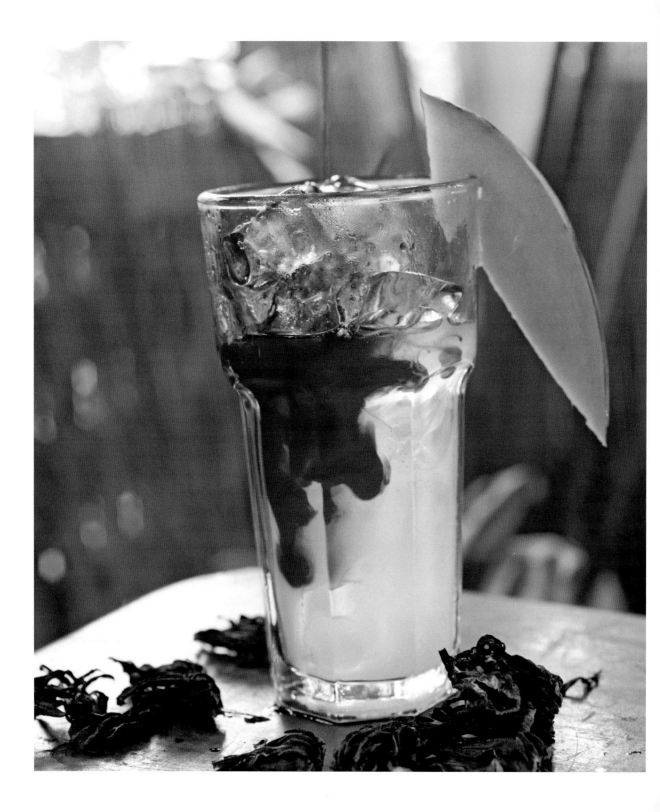

SPARKLING VITAMIN C

There are multiple sources of vitamin C. This tonic boosts ordinary grapefruit juice with a megaload of antioxidants from naturally sweet gynostemma leaves and sour hibiscus. Infusing these beauties produces an irresistible nectar, enriched with nutrients.

Makes 1–2 servings

> 1 tablespoon gynostemma tea
> 2 tablespoons hibiscus flower
> 1 cup boiling water
> 3 ounces beet juice
> 4 ounces grapefruit juice
> 3 ounces cold-pressed ginger juice
> 1 teaspoon camu camu powder
> Ice
> Sparkling water

1. Steep the gynostemma tea and hibiscus in the boiling water.

2. Allow to steep for about 15 minutes, then strain.

3. Put the tea in the fridge to cool, or wait until it's lukewarm.

4. Combine the cooled infusion, beet juice, grapefruit juice, ginger juice, and camu camu.

5. Fill glasses with ice, fill the glasses two-thirds of the way with the mixture, and top with sparkling water.

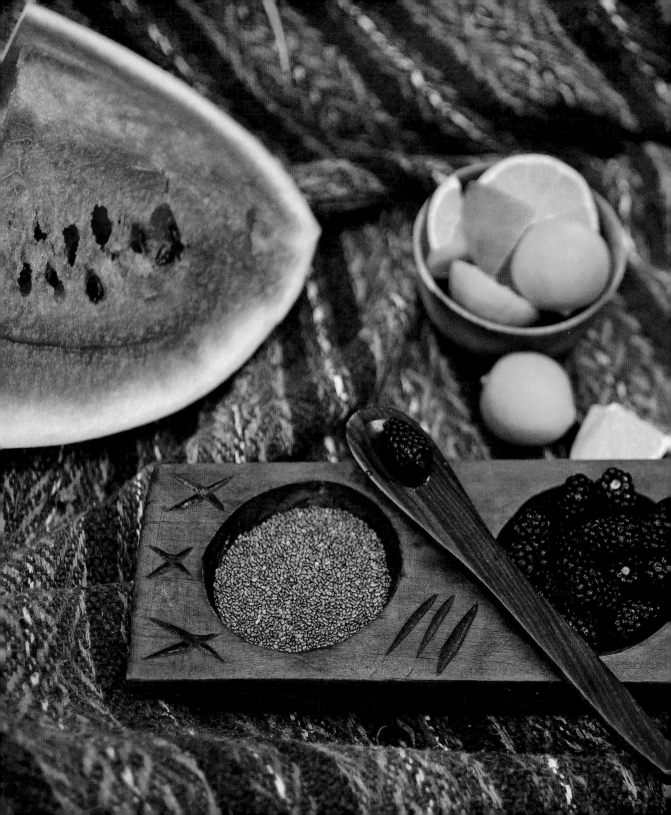

WATERMELON ALOE CHIA FRESCA

This drink is a delicious way to nourish the digestive system and the kidneys. Aloe and chia have been used for centuries to treat kidney imbalances. Once hydrated, chia transforms into a slimy substance similar to aloe. The holy slime they both share is very similar to the protective lining in our gut.

Makes 2 servings

12 ounces cold-pressed watermelon juice
8 ounces fresh aloe juice
2 tablespoons chia seeds
1 ounce lemon juice
Handful mint leaves
Ice

1. In a blender, combine the watermelon juice, aloe juice, chia seeds, and lemon juice. Pulse for a few seconds to dissolve the aloe and awaken the chia seeds.

2. Bruise the mint leaves a bit by muddling them into the ice.

3. Add the juice, and enjoy.

RHODIOLA SANGRIA SPRITZ

*This virgin probiotic-rich sangria
contains a potent tonic herb punch.
You'll feel naturally high from drinking
this exquisite compilation of herbal
boosters!*

Makes 6–8 servings

2 cups boiling water
2 black tea bags (or 2 teaspoons
   loose-leaf tea in an infuser)
2 cinnamon sticks
6 cardamom pods
½ cup coconut sugar or agave
¼ cup goji berries
Cold water as needed
3 cups fresh pomegranate juice
1 cup fresh-squeezed orange juice
¼ ounce damiana extract
½ ounce rhodiola extract
½ ounce Joy Mother Tonic (see page 131)
1 medium orange, sliced into thin rounds
1 medium lime, sliced into thin rounds
1 medium green apple, cut into
   small chunks
3 cups sparkling water
Ice

1. Pour the boiling water over the tea bags, cinnamon, and cardamom, and steep for 5 minutes. Discard the tea bags and stir in the sugar to dissolve.

2. Blend the goji berries in a high-speed blender with just enough water to make them creamy.

3. In a large jar or pitcher, combine the tea, goji berries, pomegranate juice, orange juice, damiana extract, rhodiola extract, joy mother tonic, orange slices, lime slices, and apple chunks. Refrigerate for at least 1 hour, or preferably overnight.

4. Just before serving, stir in the sparkling water. Serve in glasses over ice.

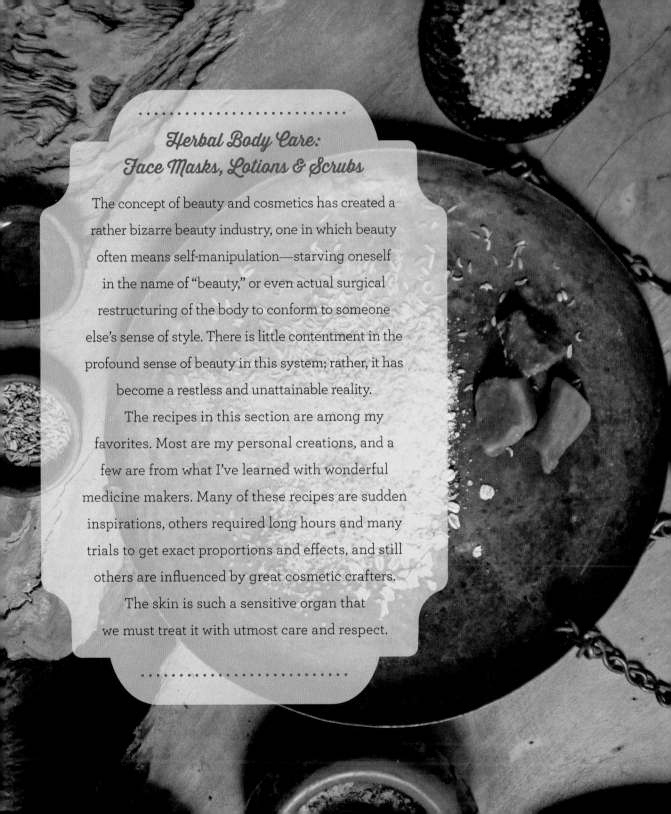

Herbal Body Care: Face Masks, Lotions & Scrubs

The concept of beauty and cosmetics has created a rather bizarre beauty industry, one in which beauty often means self-manipulation—starving oneself in the name of "beauty," or even actual surgical restructuring of the body to conform to someone else's sense of style. There is little contentment in the profound sense of beauty in this system; rather, it has become a restless and unattainable reality.

The recipes in this section are among my favorites. Most are my personal creations, and a few are from what I've learned with wonderful medicine makers. Many of these recipes are sudden inspirations, others required long hours and many trials to get exact proportions and effects, and still others are influenced by great cosmetic crafters.

The skin is such a sensitive organ that we must treat it with utmost care and respect.

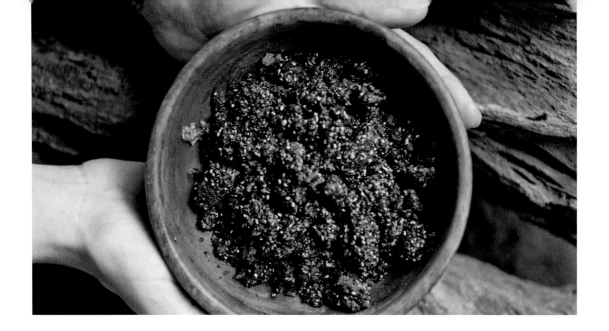

COFFEE AND RAW SUGAR SCRUB

Scrubs are a superb lymph stimulant. A vigorous scrub can help get the lymphatic system up to par, so we can purify and excrete toxins and other waste. Not much attention is usually paid to the lymphatic system. A lot of people see cleansing only as a gut detox, when in fact our lymphatic system has a great role within the elimination process. Two key ways it is activated are sweating and hands-on practices (massage, scrubbing, etc.).

5 parts raw brown sugar
3 parts ground coffee
2 parts raw coconut oil
Splash of vanilla extract

1. Mix the sugar and the coffee together.

2. Add the oil and vanilla slowly, mixing with your hands.

Basic Rules for Vibrant Skin

1. Use cruelty-free products.

2. Make all your cosmetics yourself, if possible.

3. Use vegetable and herbal sources for your ingredients.

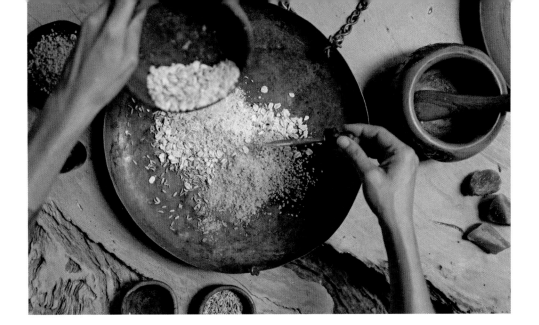

MILKY PINK SALT BATH

Heat + salt = healthy skin and lymph. Dilating the pores with a steamy bath, with the addition of exquisite salts, is a key practice to keeping vibrant skin and a purified lymphatic system.

> 4 parts Epsom salt
> 3 parts pink salt
> 2 parts oats
> 1 part hemp seeds
> Add ylang-ylang essential oil as you like.

1. Mix all ingredients together.

2. Use and enjoy as needed!

GOLDEN FACIAL SERUM

I constantly tell people to beware of oils and face cosmetics. There are way too many dirty and expensive cosmetics out there that ruin sensitive skin. If you look closely at the ingredients list of commercially prepared serums, you'll see that they are expensive combinations of chemicals that we shouldn't really put on our face. It's so easy to make your own serums that are truly good for your skin—and easy on your wallet!

    1 tablespoon jojoba oil
    2 teaspoons rose hip oil
    1 teaspoon apricot kernel oil
    4 drops calendula essential oil
    4 drops sandalwood oil
    2 drops carrot seed oil

1. Combine all ingredients, and mix well.

Skin Care Ritual

This sweet ritual results in vibrant skin. I'd recommend you do this three times per week.

1. In the morning, while you are in the shower, cover your whole body with Coffee and Raw Sugar Scrub (see page 102), then rub it into your skin with circular motions. Rinse well.

2. Nourish with Best Body Oil (see page 105) after your shower.

3. Close pores with Heart Chakra Mist (see page 106) or Queen of Hungary Water (see page 109).

4. At night, cleanse with Milky Pink Salt Bath (see page 103).

5. Follow this ritual with a light massage using Perfect Cream (see page 112).

AVOCADO AND CLAY MASK

This mask will soothe skin and clarify pores.

Makes 1 application

>   1 teaspoon bentonite clay
>   1 teaspoon fresh avocado
>   1–2 teaspoons water (or more if needed)
>   3 drops rose geranium essential oil

1. Mix the clay with the avocado, making a thick paste.

2. Add warm water slowly, making the paste smoother and smoother.

3. Mix in the essential oil.

4. Immediately apply to face and neck in a circular motion.

5. Leave for about 10–15 minutes until it hardens.

6. Remove with a washcloth soaked in hot water (hot water helps you avoid scraping your skin too much).

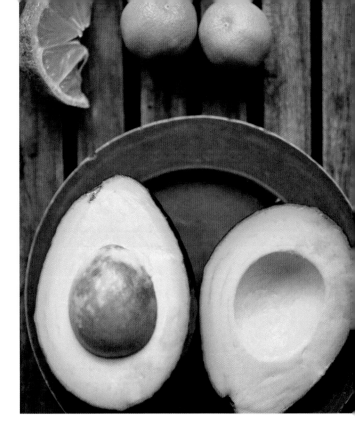

THE BEST BODY OIL

This is a decadent and nourishing body oil with a grounding and floral scent.

>   1 tablespoon avocado oil
>   2 teaspoons rose hip oil
>   1 teaspoon argan or apricot kernel oil
>   1 teaspoon jojoba oil
>   10 drops carrot seed oil
>   5 drops orange or grapefruit essential oil
>   3 drops sandalwood essential oil
>   3 drops rose geranium essential oil

1. Mix all ingredients together.

HEART CHAKRA MIST

Flower water is technically a hydrosol, yet this is quite a gratifying shortcut to installing a distillation lab. Flower waters are great to keep around for aromatherapeutic qualities, as a cooling mist, and as a source to cleanse energy. In shamanism, flower waters are used as limpias, meaning they cleanse the soul from impurities and bad energy.

> 7 parts water
> 3 parts 100 proof vodka
> 4 parts rose essential oil
> 4 parts palo santo essential oil
> 2 parts jasmine essential oil

1. Combine the water and vodka.

2. Mix the rose, palo santo, and jasmine essential oils.

3. Add the oils to the water and alcohol solution, and pour into a spray bottle.

4. Mist, and enjoy!

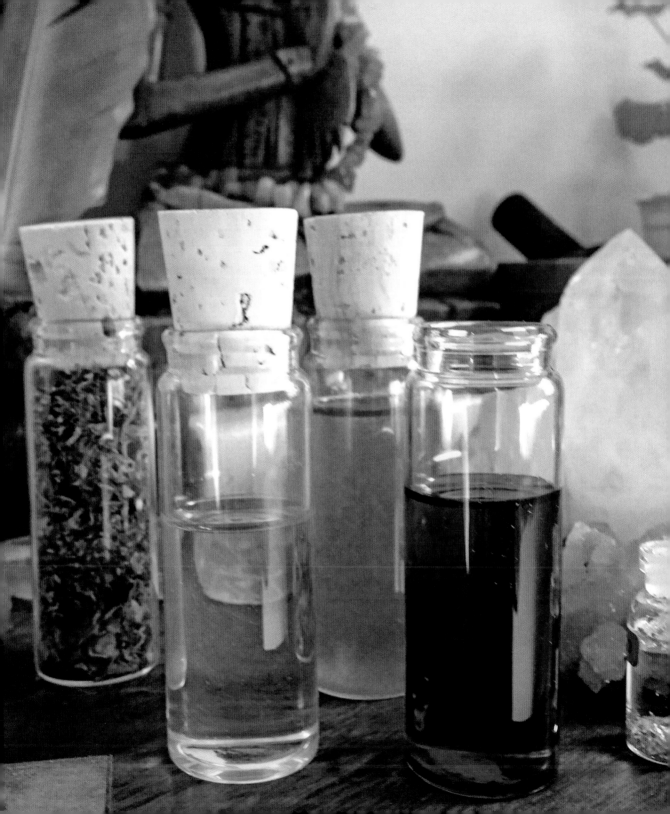

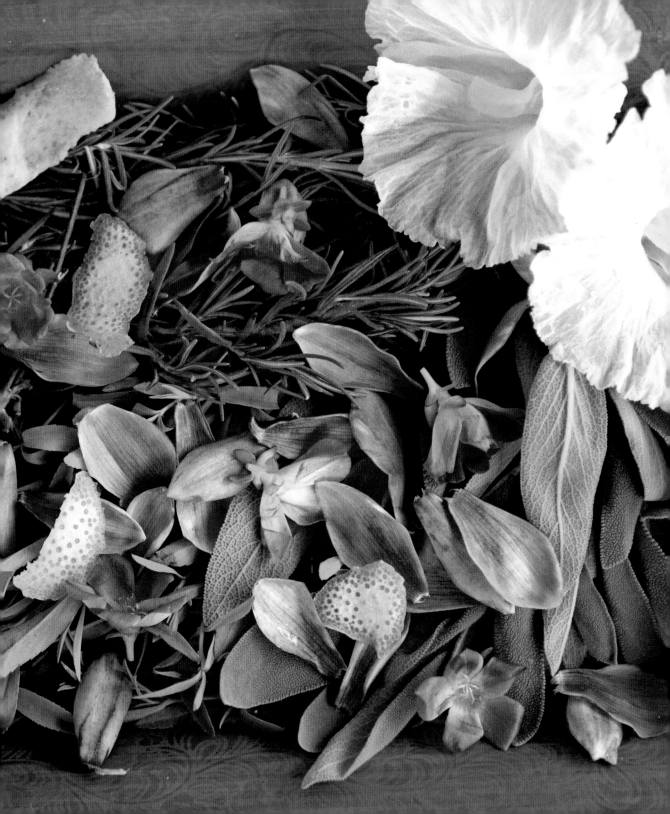

QUEEN OF HUNGARY WATER

This wonderful astringent wash has been revered for quite some time.
Legend has it that a very handsome traveling man used it to heal the queen
of Hungary of a mysterious disease. As a result, it has been a precious water
sold and marketed at very high-end places since ancient times among both
common and royal people. The good news is that you can easily make it
yourself and see rewarding effects quite quickly!

6 parts lemon balm leaf
4 parts chamomile flowers
4 parts rose petals
3 parts calendula flowers
3 parts comfrey leaf
1 part lemon peel
1 part rosemary leaf
Apple cider vinegar (amount will vary depending on the container used)
   Rose Water (see page 110) or witch hazel extract (amount will vary depending on
   the container used)
Essential oil of your choice

1. Place all the herbs in a glass jar. Add enough vinegar to cover the herbs by
   2–3 inches. Place the lid on the jar and let sit in a warm spot for 2–3 weeks.

2. Strain the herbs, and keep the liquid. For each cup of liquid, add ½–1 cup of rose
   water or witch hazel extract. If desired, you can add a drop or two of essential
   oil. Store the liquid in a glass container with a lid; it will keep indefinitely
   without refrigeration.

3. To use as a facial toner, you can apply it with a cotton ball or use it in a mister
   bottle to spray directly onto the face or over the body.

ROSE WATER

Though rose water is generally made by distillation, this method of infusion is simple and effective.

Makes 16 ounces

1½ cups witch hazel, or vodka
½ cup distilled water
3 cups fresh rosebuds (dry can work as well)

1. Mix the witch hazel extract with the distilled water.

2. Place the rosebuds in wide-mouth quart jar. Add enough of the diluted witch hazel to fill the jar.

3. Cover tightly, and let sit for 2–3 weeks in a warm, dark area.

4. Strain out the roses, reserving the liquid. Transfer the rose water to a glass container and store in a cool, dark place, where it will keep for up to a year.

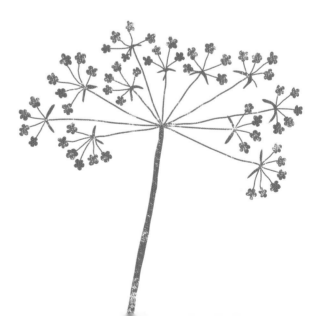

HERBAL FACIAL STEAM

A facial steam is like a sauna for the face. It draws fresh blood to the surface and purifies toxic accumulation in the epidermis. It also relieves the nasal passages while opening the skin in the face and surrounding areas. Get creative with your own recipe—you can add some of your favorite flowers to the mix.

Makes 1 treatment

> 1 part lavender flower
> 2 parts chamomile blossoms
> 2 parts calendula flowers
> 1 part rose petals

1. Bring 2–3 quarts of water to a boil in a big pot.

2. Add the flowers, and simmer for a few minutes.

3. Sit at a table in front of the pot, and drape a large thick towel over your head and the pot.

4. Place your face over the steam, inhaling and exhaling deeply.

5. The closer your head is to the pot, the hotter it will get, so be careful.

6. Spritz your face with some cool water or Heart Chakra Mist (see page 106) to close the pores back up when you are done.

THE PERFECT CREAM

This recipe is made by one of my herbal gurus, Rosemary Gladstar. This is a magnificent and decadent recipe that is relatively inexpensive, rich, and deeply nourishing. Ingredients can be varied as you like. Although it's usually recommended as a face cream, the rest of your body will surely love to be lathered with this delicious lotion.

KEEP IN MIND BEFORE STARTING:

Temperature is everything. All ingredients should be at room temperature when you begin.

Proportions. The overall proportions should roughly be 1 part water to 1 part oil. The oils should break down as approximately 2 parts liquid oil (for example, almond or apricot kernel oil) and 1 part solid oil (for example, coconut oil or cocoa butter).

Be creative! Try a small batch and feel free to substitute other carrier and essential oils to make your favorite cream. Different essential oils will lend different scents to your cream.

GROUP 1: Waters

⅔ cup distilled water, Rose Water (see page 110), or another hydrosol
⅓ cup commercially prepared aloe vera gel
1–2 drops essential oil of choice
500–1,000 IUs vitamin A (optional)
500–1,000 IUs vitamin E (optional)

GROUP 2: Oils

¾ cup carrier oil (such as apricot kernel, almond, or grapeseed); I like to combine two or three oils for their different qualities

⅓ cup solid or semisolid oil (such as coconut oil, shea butter, and/or cocoa butter)

¼ teaspoon lanolin (optional)

½–1 ounce grated beeswax (or other solid wax), for thickening

1. Combine all the elements of group 1—the distilled water or hydrosol, aloe vera gel, essential oil, and vitamins A and E (if using)—in a glass measuring cup. Whisk together. Set aside.

2. In a double boiler over very low heat, combine the elements of group 2—the carrier oil, solid or semisolid oil, lanolin (if using), and beeswax. Heat just enough to melt the solids. Stir well, and then set aside and let cool to room temperature. This takes a couple of hours. I often melt these oils and waxes the night before and then let them sit overnight. (You can hurry the process by placing the cooling mixture in the refrigerator, but keep an eye on it so it doesn't get too cold. It needs to be room temperature when you begin to emulsify.)

3. When the oil mixture has cooled to room temperature, pour it into a blender. Be sure the lid is on tightly, and turn on the blender at its highest speed (a high-speed blender works best). Slowly, in a thin, steady drizzle, pour in the water mixture, aiming the stream of liquid into the center vortex of the whirling oil mixture. Be sure to do this steadily and slowly, so that the water molecules can emulsify and blend with the oil molecules.

4. When you have added most of the water mixture to the oils and the cream has begun to thicken, listen to the blender and watch the cream. When the blender coughs and chokes, and the cream looks thick and white, like buttercream frosting, turn off the blender. If there is water remaining in the glass cup, you can slowly try to add a little more, beating it in by hand with a spoon, but don't overbeat! Be patient: the cream will thicken as it sets.

5. When it has cooled, package your cream in clean, dry glass jars. The cream, even though it has no preservatives in it, will last for several months if stored in a cool location; it doesn't need to be refrigerated.

TIP:

Aloe vera gel will make the cream heavier than if you were to use only water. Aloe is very healing and moisturizing to the skin, yet it's up to you how heavy you'd like this cream. Beware of using fresh aloe for this—it expires quickly, making the cream go bad within a week or so of being made.

TIP:

This recipe is a bit challenging, as you are attempting to emulsify water and oil. Follow the recipe closely. If it doesn't turn out the first time, don't be discouraged. Let it sit in the blender until the liquid and oils separate (usually just a few hours or overnight); then pour off the liquid and try again. If it doesn't come together on the first try, it generally seems to blend on the second. Or just leave it as is—pour it into a bottle and simply shake well before using.

JUICE SENSORIUM

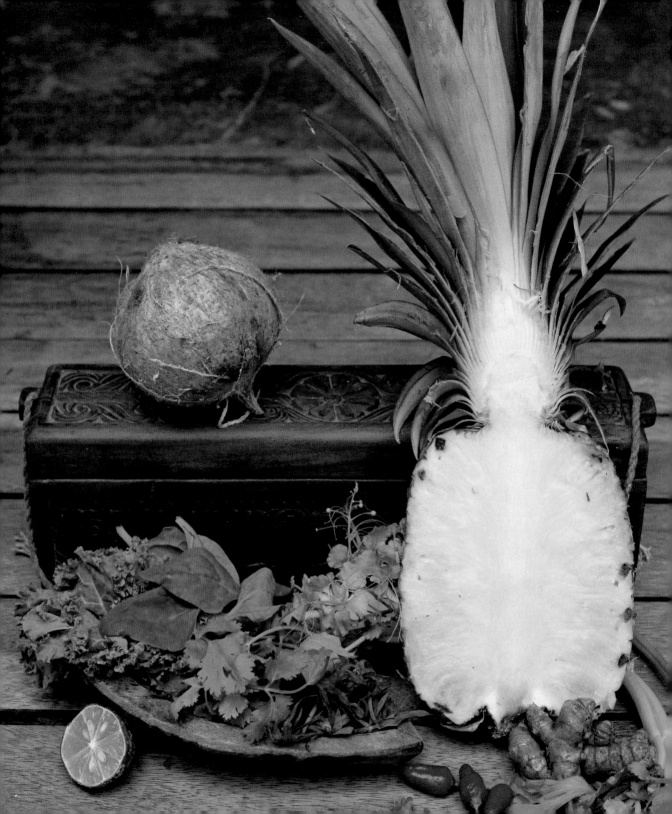

The Juice Sensorium contains recipes that have a little more than the usual kitchen prep work, with considerably more influence from tonic herbs. Each section is broken down into general categories based on the body systems. This can help you guide yourself when you desire to make something to target specific issues that may be affecting you. These categories will also give you an idea of what body systems you are targeting simultaneously.

Within each section I describe a "mother extract" for that category, a blend of herbs in extract (tincture) form that you can keep in your kitchen cabinet. There are six base master tonics you can use with your juices, teas, and smoothies. Study the effects of these tonics and see what you'd change in them for you to formulate even a better combination each time you craft it.

Don't be intimidated—herbal extracts are so easy to make. You'll love the process, and even when you think you made a little bit, it's still a large enough amount to have around at home to share with friends and family.

BEAUTY TONICS:
ANTI-AGING AND DETOX

Main body components:
Skin, liver, gall bladder

These tonics cover:
Anti-aging, detox, cleansers

JOY TONICS:
HAPPINESS AND BLISS

Main body components:
Brain, psyche, heart

These tonics cover: Mental balance,
happiness, circulation, aphrodisiacs

ENERGY TONICS:
EUPHORIC AND STRENGTHENING

Main body components: Reproductive
system, muscles, immune system

These tonics cover: Strengthening, euphoria,
sustainable energy tonics

RELAXING TONICS:
DESTRESS AND UNWIND

Main body components:
Nervous system, respiratory system

These tonics cover:
Calming, destressing, unwinders

NOURISHING TONICS:
REPLENISH AND REJUVENATE

Main body components:
Stomach, intestines, kidneys

These tonics cover: Replenishing,
rejuvenation, mineralization

SPIRIT TONICS:
CLARITY AND BALANCE

Main body components: Mind, body, spirit

These tonics cover: Meditation, clarity,
balance, lucid dreaming

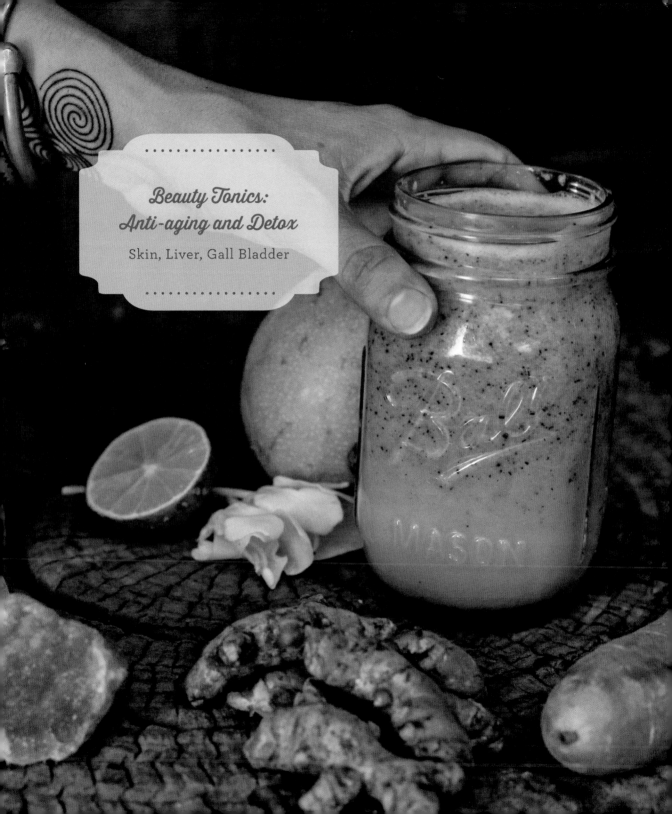

Beauty Tonics:
Anti-aging and Detox

Skin, Liver, Gall Bladder

SKIN DETOX

Makes 1–2 servings

1 cup boiling water
1 tablespoon calendula flowers
1 tablespoon gotu kola leaves
8 ounces orange juice
4 ounces grapefruit juice
2 ounces burdock root juice
1 teaspoon turmeric powder
1 teaspoon lemon juice

1. Add the boiling water to the calendula flowers and gotu kola leaves. Allow the mixture to infuse for about 15 minutes. Strain the herbs and keep the water.

2. Mix the orange, grapefruit, burdock root juices together.

3. Combine both mixtures, then add the turmeric and lemon juice.

4. Shake well, and enjoy!

CELLULITE BLASTER

Ahh . . . the mysteries of cellulite. First, it is not permanent. Second, an essential key to its treatment is exercise. By combining fat-burning tonics with specific exercises that target the dimpled areas, you'll be able to bust it out of you within a reasonable time. This tonic is recommended in conjunction with an alkaline diet and regular exercise for optimum effects.

Makes 1 serving

> 6 ounces dark leafy green mix juice (kale, collards, chard, parsley)
> 2 ounces cold-pressed ginger juice
> 2 ounces fresh turmeric root juice
> 1 teaspoon lemon juice
> 1 teaspoon spirulina
> ½ teaspoon garcinia cambogia powder
> Juice of ½ green apple (optional)

Note: Garcinia has been widely used in the rainforests of Thailand and in South America primarily for detox, and now it is popularly used a weight-loss miracle. The acid within the fruit, HCA, inhibits the formation of fatty acids, and therefore less fat is available to the cells to be stored by the body.

1. Mix the juices together. Add the spirulina and garcinia cambogia, and shake well until the powder is dissolved.

2. If the juice is too bitter for you, add the juice of ½ of a green apple.

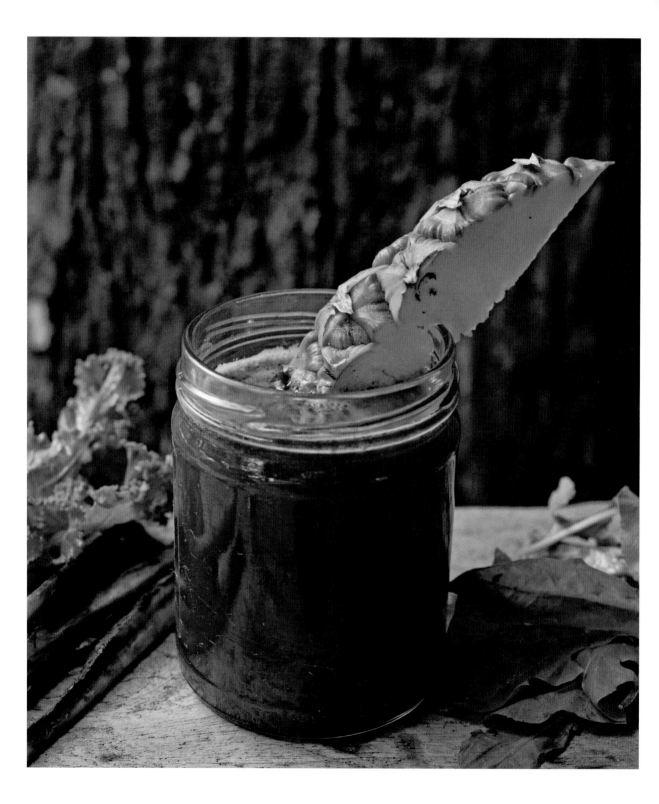

LOVE HANDLES

This is a pungent fat-burning formula using some of the rainforest's finest tonics to relieve stagnation and slow gut metabolism. It is a potent detoxifying juice tonic known for its sustainable weight-loss support.

Makes 1 serving

10 ounces pineapple juice
4 ounces kale juice
1 ounce dandelion
1 ounce parsley
½ teaspoon cha de bugre extract or powder
½ teaspoon garcinia cambogia extract or powder

Note: Cha de bugre has long been a popular weight-loss product that has been marketed as a diuretic and appetite suppressant. It is believed to help prevent or reduce fatty deposits and cellulite.

1. Mix all ingredients together in a shaker, and shake well.

MASTER DETOXIFIER: DETOX SHOT

This tonic is a detoxifying powerhouse that will drain out toxic accumulation from the liver, blood, and gut. Spirulina and dandelion draw out inflammation, heavy metals, and bacteria, bringing next-level mineralization to the entire body.

Makes 3 servings

1 tablespoon spirulina
½ ounce lemon juice
Handful dandelion greens
8 ounces fresh coconut water

Extra Boost: ½ teaspoon Beauty Mother Tonic (see page 125)

1. Blend all ingredients together, and serve in short glasses.

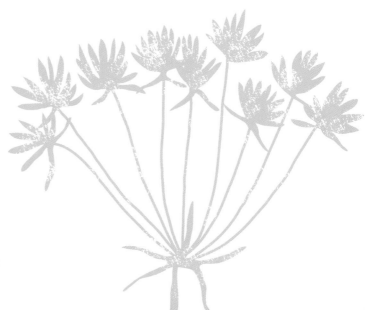

BEAUTY MOTHER TONIC

This is an everyday miracle tonic for glowing skin, bright eyes, and a healthy liver.

Makes one "mother tonic"

2 parts turmeric
2 parts gotu kola
2 parts dried burdock
2 parts dried mangosteen
1 part dried calendula flowers
100 proof vodka or rum (amount will vary)
Lemon peel, fresh, not dried*

1. Place the herbs in a wide-mouth jar, to fill about one-third of the jar.

2. Cover the herbs in vodka and allow them to soak in the liquid.

3. Press the herbs down with your hand or a tool. A general rule of thumb is that if you have about 1–2 inches of liquid going over the herbs, then you have a great ratio! If the herbs still look dry, add a little more liquid.

4. Add a handful of fresh slices of lemon peel to the mix.

5. To prevent rust, cover the jar with a fine cloth or plastic wrap, and place the lid on top.

6. Place in a cool, dry place, and allow 3–4 weeks for the herbs to macerate in the liquid. Shake the jar every other day.

7. Strain the liquid into a clean jar, and press the herbs in a fine-mesh cloth. Keep pressing until the herbs are basically dried out.

8. Store the tonic in a cool place, and prevent exposure to light.

Recommended dosage: 1 teaspoon, 2–3 times per day, directly or in your choice of juice, smoothie, or tea.

---

* Using fresh lemon peel will give an extra punch to the flavor and a higher antioxidant count.

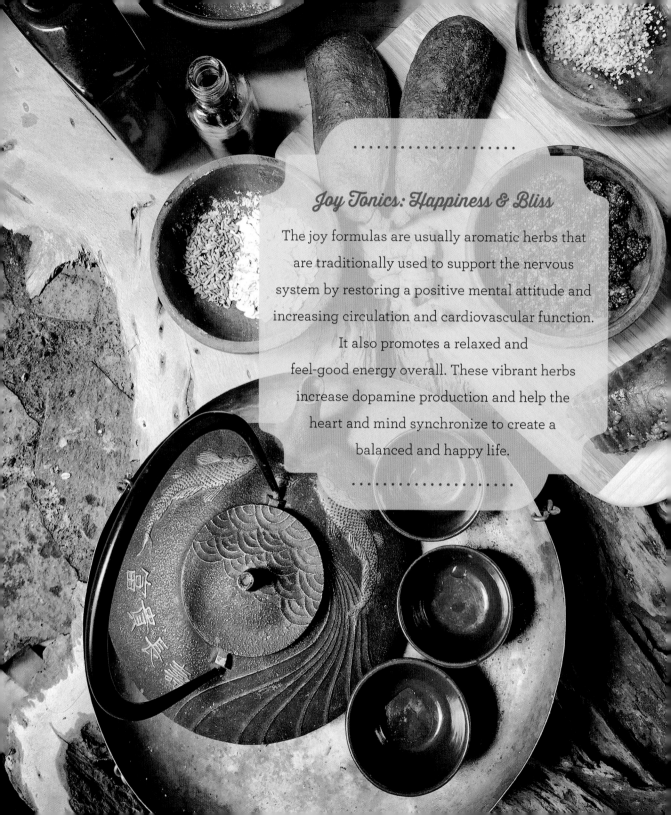

Joy Tonics: Happiness & Bliss

The joy formulas are usually aromatic herbs that are traditionally used to support the nervous system by restoring a positive mental attitude and increasing circulation and cardiovascular function. It also promotes a relaxed and feel-good energy overall. These vibrant herbs increase dopamine production and help the heart and mind synchronize to create a balanced and happy life.

DOPAMINE BOOSTER

Dopamine is a neurotransmitter, one of those chemicals that is responsible for transmitting signals between the nerve cells (neurons) of the brain. Very few neurons actually make dopamine. This holy chemical is responsible for our "Aha" moments, and generally insightful moments in which we connect the dots on what seemed vague before.

Makes 1–2 servings

2 tablespoons cacao powder
1 cup almond milk (see page 74)
1 teaspoon coconut oil
1 frozen banana
1 date
1 teaspoon St. John's wort extract
½ teaspoon albizzia extract
1 teaspoon rhodiola powder or extract
Ice as needed for consistency
1 teaspoon cacao nibs

Omega-3 Fatty Acids

An essential component to shaking off a bout of depression is to drink your omega-3 fatty acids. The brain is nearly 60% fat by weight, and much of that fat consists of omega-3 fatty acids, which serve as structural components of the brain's cells and tissues. My favorite plant-based sources are flax seed oil, chia seed oil, walnut oil, and radish seed oil.

1. Blend all ingredients except the cacao nibs together until creamy.

2. Add the nibs, and pulse briefly to mix, to keep nice crunchy bites in your smoothie.

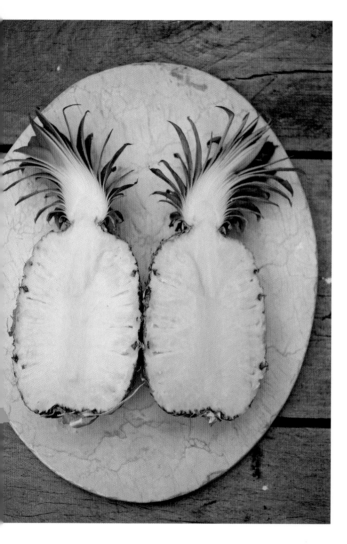

GOOD MOOD TONIC

This tonic contains a tasty mix of herbs known to shake sadness away from your mind and heart. These herbs have been used for centuries to shake off depression and help relieve the mind from negative patterns.

Makes 2 servings

> 8 ounces green apple juice
> 12 ounces pineapple juice
> 1–2 teaspoons St. John's wort extract
> 3 drops lemon balm essential oil
> ⅓ teaspoon flax oil
> Fresh lemon balm leaves (optional)
> Ice
> Sparkling water

1. Mix the green apple and pineapple juices.

2. Add the St. John's wort extract, lemon balm essential oil, and flax oil.

3. If you are able to find fresh lemon balm, bruise the leaves into a glass with ice.

4. Pour the juice and tonics into the glass with ice, and add sparkling water to the top.

APHRODISIAC COCKTAIL

This "cocktail" is a floral and awakening tonic known to bring circulation to the heart and reproductive organs. It will awaken the sacral chakra and bring circulation to the pelvic area.

Makes 2 servings

1 tablespoon catuaba
1 teaspoon muira puama
1 teaspoon damiana
2½ cups warm water, divided use
½ cup goji berries
14 ounces pomegranate juice
6 ounces black grape juice
Ice cubes
½ sweet orange

1. Bring the catuaba, muira puama, and damiana to a boil in 2 cups of the water. Simmer for 15 minutes.

2. In a separate container, soak the goji berries in the remaining ½ cup of water.

3. In the blender, add the pomegranate juice, grape juice, and the hydrated goji berries with any remaining berry water. Blend until smooth.

4. Once the infusion is ready, strain out the herbs, and allow it to cool down. Add the infusion to the fruit juices, and blend until smooth.

5. Pour into glasses filled with ice. Press by hand about 1 teaspoon of orange juice into each glass. Enjoy!

HEART CHAKRA COCKTAIL

Dragon fruit and figs have been used since ancient times as cardiovascular tonics and heart openers. Energetically they have been known by healers to open the upper body's subtle system, and they are an essential source for upper body circulation.

Note: Dragon fruit, also known as pitahaya, is considered a heart healer by many Central American tribes. In Mexico there is a dance known as La Flor de Pitahaya that is said to pay homage to the Queen of the Night. In Costa Rica and other parts of Central America, it is a staple fruit revered for its potent nutrients and mystical energy.

Makes 2 servings

½ cup frozen strawberries
½ cup dragon fruit
1–2 ounces beet juice
1 teaspoon of Joy Mother Tonic (see page 131)
1 teaspoon coconut sugar or choice of sweetener
3 drops jasmine essential oil

1. Combine the strawberries, dragon fruit, and beet juice in a blender, and blend until smooth.

2. Mix in the tonic.

3. Add the coconut sugar and essential oil, and blend.

JOY MOTHER TONIC

This is a great base tonic for feeling ecstatic and a general therapeutic formula for your brain and reproductive system. I combine these to feel circulation at both extremes of the body. With this tonic you'll feel the base chakra and the crown chakra nourished, which naturally will bring a sense of joy.

Makes 1 "Mother Tonic"

> 3 parts dried rhodiola
> 2 parts dried St. John's wort
> 2 parts dried green coffee bean
> 2 parts dried ginkgo
> 1 part dried ginger
> 100 proof vodka or rum

1. Place the herbs in a wide-mouth jar, to fill about one-third of the jar.

2. Cover the herbs in vodka and allow them to soak in the liquid slowly.

3. Press the herbs down with your hand or a tool. A general rule of thumb is that if you have about 1–2 inches of liquid going over the herbs, then you have a great ratio! If the herbs still look dry, add a little more liquid.

4. To prevent rust, cover the jar with a fine cloth or plastic wrap, and place the lid on top.

5. Place in a cool, dry place, and allow 3–4 weeks for the herbs to macerate in the liquid. Shake the jar every other day.

6. Strain the liquid into a clean jar, and press the herbs in a fine-mesh cloth. Keep pressing until the herbs are basically dried out.

7. Store the tonic in a cool place, and prevent exposure to light.

Recommended dosage: 1–2 teaspoons, 2–3 times per day, or as needed.

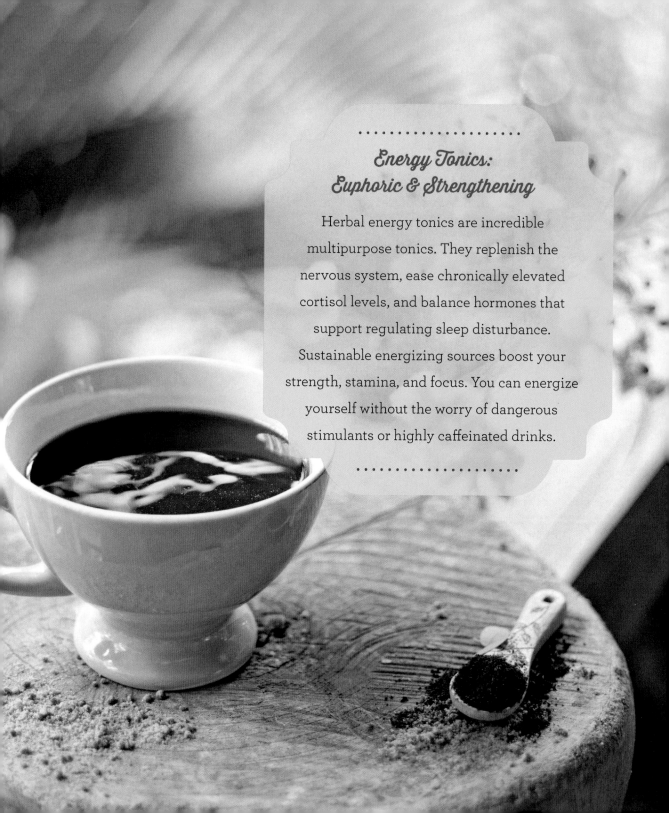

Energy Tonics: Euphoric & Strengthening

Herbal energy tonics are incredible multipurpose tonics. They replenish the nervous system, ease chronically elevated cortisol levels, and balance hormones that support regulating sleep disturbance. Sustainable energizing sources boost your strength, stamina, and focus. You can energize yourself without the worry of dangerous stimulants or highly caffeinated drinks.

GET HIGH

A sustainably energizing coffee alternative, green coffee bean and guayusa energize you just enough to feel awake throughout the day. Their mineralizing power regulates blood sugar, reducing stress and increasing muscle and nerve function.

Note: Guayusa is traditionally used by certain tribal peoples in Peru as a night tonic, to help facilitate lucid dreaming. Shamans take it at 3 a.m. to induce a lucid state, which is said to help you stay awake in the dream.

Makes 1 serving

> 2 tablespoons guayusa leaf
> 6–8 ounces almost-boiling water
> 2 tablespoons matcha
> ½ teaspoon Energy Mother Tonic (see page 139)
> Stevia or honey
> Almond milk (optional, see page 74)

1. In a teapot, steep the guayusa in ½ cup hot water (almost boiling).

2. In a cup, add the matcha powder, and pour ½ cup of hot water into it. With a whisk, mix it well until it's completely dissolved.

3. Add the guayusa infusion into the matcha, and add the energy tonic.

4. Add stevia and almond milk to taste.

MIDNIGHT

This tonic is a delicious approach to coffee that provides energy but prevents an adrenal crash. Many of us love a frothy cup of coffee in the morning. And even though we know that it's not healthy to drink too much of it, we still keep on doing it. Here is an alternative that prevents the adrenals from drying up and cramping, while enhancing immunity.

Makes 1 serving

1 teaspoon chaga
2 tablespoons ground coffee
6–8 ounces almost-boiling water
4–6 ounces nut milk of choice (see page 74)
Sweetener of choice

Boost it! Add 1 teaspoon of roasted dandelion root for an extra healthy punch.

1. In a French press, add the chaga and coffee. Pour in the water, and allow it to steep for about 5 minutes before pouring it into a cup.

2. Add milk and sweetener to taste, and enjoy!

Note: To make this noncaffeinated, simmer 1 tablespoon of chaga and 2 cups of water in a pot for about 15 minutes. Strain and enjoy!

IMMUNITY SHOT

The best kind of herbs to drink are immune boosters and adaptogens.
Together, they support white blood cell production and all major organs while
balancing, restoring, and protecting the body as a whole.

Makes 2 servings

> 1 teaspoon turmeric powder
> 1 teaspoon lemon juice
> 1–2 teaspoons Energy Mother Tonic (see page 139)
> 1 teaspoon cat's claw powder
> 1 teaspoon coconut oil
> 1 teaspoon raw honey or agave
> Water

1. Mix all ingredients together, and shoot!

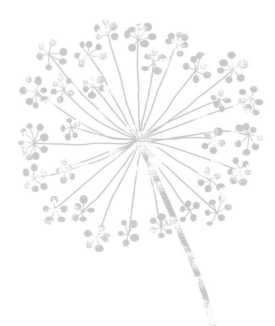

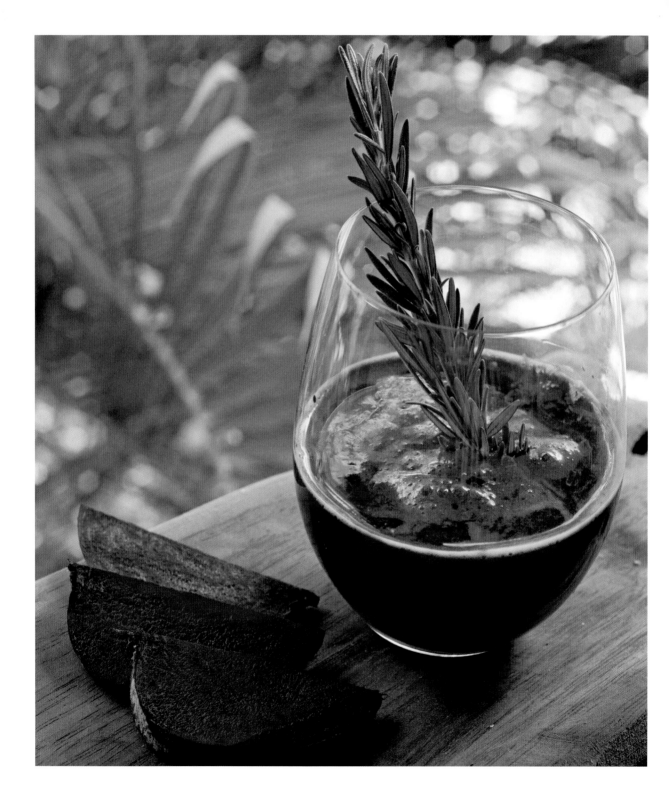

BRAIN TONIC

A bright and sweet tonic with a refreshing twist to alert the mind. Brain tonics energize the brain by boosting memory and sharpening focus.

Makes 1 serving

> 4 ounces beet juice
> 8 ounces pomegranate juice
> 1 ounce lemon juice
> 1 teaspoon Energy Mother Tonic (see page 139)
> Rosemary sprig

1. Mix all ingredients, except the rosemary, in a shaker. Shake well.

2. Strain into a glass, stand the rosemary in it, and enjoy.

COLDS COCKTAIL

This is one of my absolute favorite tonic drinks to kick any cold and feel good. The combination of these ingredients is delightful, and you'll be surprised at how much you love these immune-enhancing ingredients together. You'll crave it even if you are not under the weather!

Makes 1 serving

1 ounce ginger juice
1 ounce lemon juice
½ ounce garlic juice
1 ounce turmeric
Pinch cayenne
Pinch black pepper
Pinch Himalayan pink salt
½ ounce apple cider vinegar
8 ounces hot water or chilled coconut water, depending on if you want a hot or cold drink

1. Combine the ginger, lemon, and garlic juices.

2. Add the juice mixture, turmeric, cayenne, black pepper, salt, and vinegar to the water, and mix.

3. Sip slowly for the best effect.

ENERGY MOTHER TONIC

3 parts dried ginkgo
2 parts dried gotu kola
3 parts dried rhodiola
1 part dried guayusa
100 proof vodka or rum

Makes one "mother tonic"

1. Place all herbs in a wide-mouth jar, to fill about a one-third of the jar.

2. Cover the herbs in vodka, and allow them to soak in the liquid slowly.

3. Press the herbs down with your hand or a tool. A general rule of thumb is that if you have about 1–2 inches of liquid over the herbs, then you have a great ratio! If the herbs still look dry, add a little more liquid.

4. To prevent rust, cover the jar with a fine cloth or plastic wrap, and place the lid on top.

5. Place in a cool, dry place, and allow 3–4 weeks for the herbs to macerate in the liquid. Shake the jar every other day.

6. Strain the liquid into a clean jar, and press the herbs in a fine-mesh cloth. Keep pressing until the herbs are basically dried out.

7. Store the tonic in a cool place, and prevent exposure to light.

Recommended dosage: 1–2 teaspoons, 2–3 times per day, or as needed.

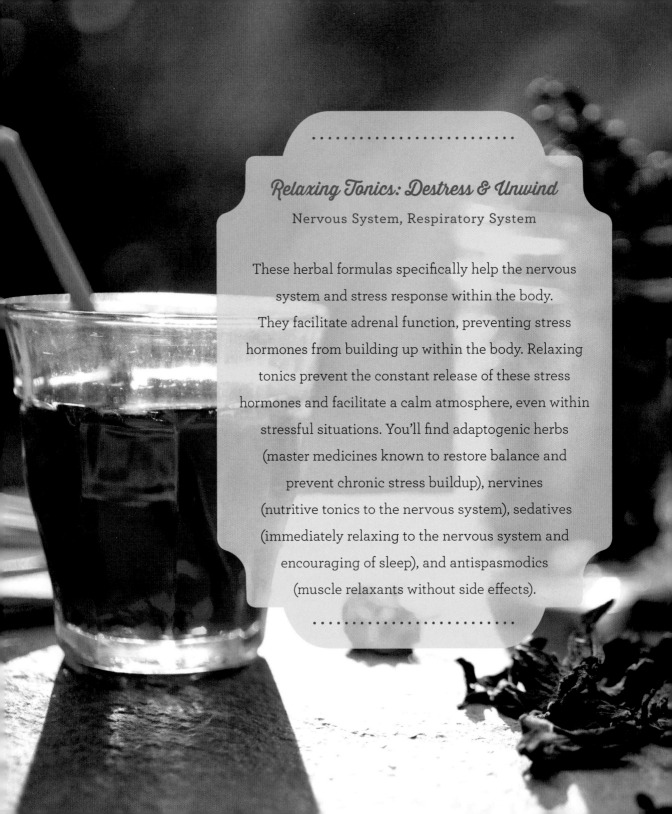

Relaxing Tonics: Destress & Unwind

Nervous System, Respiratory System

These herbal formulas specifically help the nervous system and stress response within the body. They facilitate adrenal function, preventing stress hormones from building up within the body. Relaxing tonics prevent the constant release of these stress hormones and facilitate a calm atmosphere, even within stressful situations. You'll find adaptogenic herbs (master medicines known to restore balance and prevent chronic stress buildup), nervines (nutritive tonics to the nervous system), sedatives (immediately relaxing to the nervous system and encouraging of sleep), and antispasmodics (muscle relaxants without side effects).

ADAPTOGENIC CHILLER

Adaptogens are a particular class of miracle superherbs granted their name because of their distinctive ability to "adapt" their function according to your body's needs. An adaptogen does not have a specific action, nor does it target a certain body region; rather, it benefits the body as a whole, being able to respond to any influence or stressor that it needs to.

Makes 1–2 servings

2 teaspoons schisandra berries
1 teaspoon reishi powder
1 teaspoon chaga powder
3½ cups water, divided use
¼ cup hibiscus flowers
1 scoop tamarind paste
Stevia leaf or honey
3 drops rose geranium essential oil
Ice

1. Simmer the schisandra, reishi, and chaga in 2 cups of the water.

2. Add 1 cup of boiling water to the hibiscus. Some hibiscus flowers don't release their intense color and flavor unless simmered. First try just adding boiling water to the flowers; if the potent fuchsia color isn't released, simmer it for 5 minutes. Then strain the flowers.

3. In about ½ cup of warm water, dissolve the tamarind paste. Stay. Blend the tamarind and the hibiscus water together, making a tart juice.

4. Strain the reishi, schisandra, and chaga, and once the liquid has cooled, add it to the hibiscus and tamarind mix.

5. Blend, and add stevia to taste.

6. Add the rose geranium essential oil, and pour the mixture into a glass over ice.

RELAXING KAVA MOJITO

Prevent chronically elevated cortisol levels generated by overstressing and overworking with this kava "cocktail." There is no need to burn your adrenals and kill your digestive tract with badly chosen foods and anxious behavior. Sit back and relax a bit. Enjoy this uplifting drink after a long day.

Makes 1 serving

½ fresh lime, cut into 4 wedges
2–3 tablespoons of truly raw sugar* or agave
Handful fresh mint
Ice
2–3 tablespoons kava kava extract
4 ounces sparkling water

1. Put the lime wedges into glass, then add the raw sugar and muddle. Squish everything together to release the lime juice.

2. Put the mint leaves in one hand and clap. This bruises the leaves and releases their flavor. Add the leaves to the glass.

3. Half-fill the glass with ice, and pour in the kava kava extract.

4. Top it off with about 4 ounces sparkling water, and mix with a long spoon.

5. Enjoy your cocktail!

---

* Also known as jaggery. If you are unable to find it, use agave.

STRESS RELIEF MILK

Pause and think for a minute. What is the true reason you are stressed? Strip away all the distractions and stories in your life, and sit with the authentic self that remains. This version of yourself doesn't have to think or dream; it simply is at peace in the present moment. It lives above the fray, totally untouched by the war of opposites. Stop seeking, sit with yourself in meditation, and witness the vibrancy of the empty space within your mind.

Note: When we are stressed, our brain sends a signal to the entire body, disrupting the body's metabolic balance. Stress is a state of threatened homeostasis, which means we are voluntarily threatening our cells' survival.

Makes 2 servings

2 teaspoons milky oats
16 ounces water
2 teaspoons chamomile flowers
1 teaspoons lavender flowers
Ice (optional)
Hemp milk to taste*

Note: Boost it with an adaptogen! Add 1 teaspoon rhodiola extract to enhance the destressing qualities. Rhodiola is known to be a great support for post-traumatic stress, as well as chronic stress in general.

1. In a pan, simmer the milky oats in the water for 10 minutes.

2. Add the chamomile and lavender, and simmer for an additional 10 minutes.

3. Filter out the herbs using a strainer or a teapot.

4. If you'd like this chilled, wait for it to cool down and add ice.

5. Add the milk to the tea, and enjoy!

---

* To make your own hemp milk: blend ¼ cup hemp seeds and with ¾ cup water. Filter the milk with a cheesecloth, and add sweetener to taste.

HEAD AID COCKTAIL

Headaches are triggered by imbalances in the stomach and intestines. Usually what happens is that your veins get clogged with toxins and thickened blood, causing poor circulation to build up and create pain. A backed-up digestive system, with poorly filtered blood and a side of stress, immediately causes a headache. Headaches can easily become a chronic issue if you don't take care of them properly. Unlike a migraine, a headache is not a neurological condition, yet if we don't watch what kind of food we intake or what tendency is causing the symptoms, headaches can surely become a chronic issue.

Makes 1 serving

> 10 ounces coconut water
> 6 ounces watermelon juice
> 1 teaspoon feverfew extract
> 1 teaspoon meadowsweet extract
> ½ teaspoon skullcap extract
> 2–3 drops lavender essential oil

1. Mix the coconut water and watermelon juice. Add the feverfew, meadowsweet, and skullcap.

2. Add the lavender essential oil. Mix well.

3. If the extract tastes too strong to you, add a little more coconut water and watermelon juice.

RELAX MOTHER TONIC

Makes 1 "mother tonic"

3 parts dried passionflower
3 parts dried ashwagandha
2 parts dried kava kava
2 parts dried milky oats
100 proof vodka or rum

1. Place the herbs in a wide-mouth jar, to fill about one-third of the jar.

2. Cover the herbs in vodka and allow them to soak in the liquid slowly.

3. Press the herbs down with your hand or a tool. A general rule of thumb is that if you have about 1–2 inches of liquid over the herbs, then you have a great ratio! If the herbs still look dry, add a little more liquid.

4. To prevent rust, cover the jar with a fine cloth or plastic wrap, and place the lid on top.

5. Place in a cool, dry place, and allow 3–4 weeks for the herbs to macerate in the liquid. Shake the jar every other day.

6. Strain the liquid into a clean jar, and press the herbs in a fine-mesh cloth. Keep pressing until the herbs are basically dried out.

7. Store the tonic in a cool place, and prevent exposure to light.

Recommended dosage: 1–2 teaspoons, 2–3 times per day, or as needed.

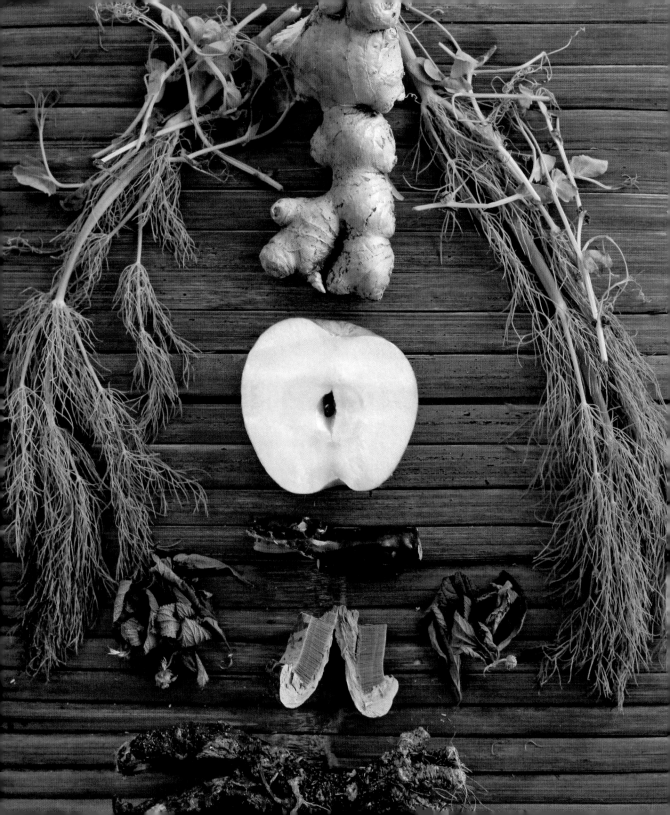

HEALTHY LUNGS TONIC TEA

Osha and schisandra are herbs that naturally moisten the lungs. They are highly aromatic as well as astringent. These herbs help to improve respiratory efficiency, moisten the respiratory membranes, clear the lungs of phlegm and toxins, and help maintain the immunocompetence of the respiratory system.

   3 parts osha root
   4 parts schisandra berries
   2 parts ginger
   9 parts water
   1 part fennel seed
   Stevia leaf or honey

1. Boil the osha, schisandra, and ginger together in the water for about 45 minutes.

2. Toward the end of the simmering process, add the fennel seeds.

3. Strain out the herbs.

4. Add stevia leaves and allow to steep for 10 minutes, or add honey to taste.

5. The tonic tea preserves very well in the fridge. Keep a jar in the fridge to drink chilled or to reheat.

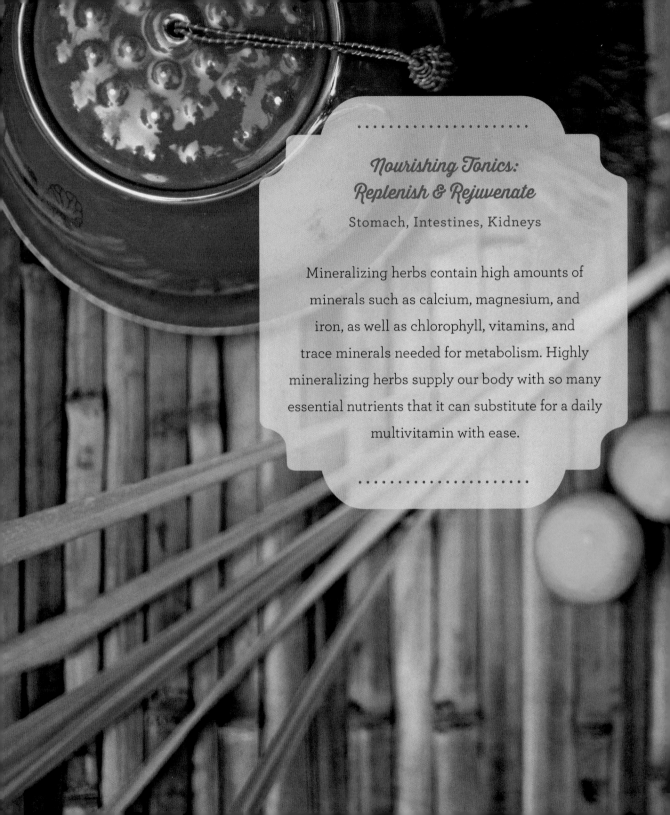

Nourishing Tonics:
Replenish & Rejuvenate

Stomach, Intestines, Kidneys

Mineralizing herbs contain high amounts of minerals such as calcium, magnesium, and iron, as well as chlorophyll, vitamins, and trace minerals needed for metabolism. Highly mineralizing herbs supply our body with so many essential nutrients that it can substitute for a daily multivitamin with ease.

PROTEIN TONIC

There are so many myths about protein. Proteins are basically huge strings of amino acids, all delicately formed to provide our bodies with support, energy, and sustenance. Fat and carbs do the same, just in different ways. Protein builds our muscles, fuels our brains, keeps our skin and hair healthy, and keeps our organs running properly. It triggers neurotransmitters in the brain to improve our mood, lower our blood sugar, and even help us focus. Protein is an important nutrient, but you don't need a tub of whey protein or a piece of chicken to get your fill.

Food for thought: Cows and gorillas grow big and strong from eating nothing but plants. Considering that a cow needs nothing more than grass to grow big and strong, why should we think any differently for ourselves? The good news is, you don't have to graze like cattle or be a gorilla to have access to nature's finest sources of protein. It's much simpler than you think, considering that so many veggies and herbs contain these essential nutrients.

Makes 2–3 servings

1 scoop almond butter
2 tablespoons hemp seeds
½ cup coconut meat (about ½ a coconut)
1½ cups coconut water
1 teaspoon spirulina
1 teaspoon mesquite
1 teaspoon ashwagandha
1 teaspoon vanilla extract
2 cups ice
Choice of sweetener (maple or agave; optional)

1. Blend all ingredients, except for the ice and sweetener, together until creamy.

2. Add the ice, and blend until frosty. Taste and sweeten as you like.

UNBLOATER

Make your own digestive bitters! Bitters, bitters, bitters! The key to preventing a bloated stomach is to have bitters 30 minutes before your meals. Bitters set the stage for perfectly balanced pH and enzymatic response for food to arrive and be efficiently broken down. In addition to dandelion's bitterness, the aromatics from the fennel, ginger, and orange will also help with that uncomfortable post-dessert bloat with carminative power. They can help relieve excess acid in the stomach, too.

Makes 1 serving

> 3 parts Oregon grape root
> 3 parts dandelion root
> 2 part orange peel
> 1 part fennel seed
> 1 part ginger root
> 100 proof vodka

1. Fill one-third of a jar with the herbs.

2. Pour vodka over the herbs and fill to the very top of the jar. Be sure the herb mixture is completely covered.

3. Label the jar with the name of the herbs, date, alcohol strength, and parts used. Allow to extract for 4–6 weeks, shaking the jar often.

4. Strain the herb with cheesecloth or a fine-mesh cloth, and squeeze any remaining liquid in the herb back into the extract.

Recommended dosage: 1 teaspoon before meals.

ANTI-ALLERGIC COCKTAIL

Although there are innumerable allergies out there, it's safe to say that if you target the liver, you'll be able to beat them—or at least ameliorate some of their side effects. If you maximize your gut health with an alkaline diet and detoxify the liver with herbal remedies like this concoction, you'll be more likely to avoid allergy suffering altogether.

Makes 1 serving

> 2 cups water
> 2 teaspoons nettle leaf
> 2 teaspoons burdock root
> 2 teaspoons chanca piedra leaf
> 12 ounces fresh grapefruit juice
> 1 tablespoon echinacea root extract
> Fresh orange peel
> Cayenne
> Ice

1. Boil the water and add the nettles, burdock, and chanca piedra. Simmer for about 15 minutes until about half of the water has evaporated.

2. Allow the infusion to cool. Once it's cooled, add 2 ounces of the liquid into the grapefruit juice. Reserve the extra for another use.

3. Add the echinacea extract.

4. Slice three long orange peel strips, and muddle the peel and a pinch of cayenne on ice.

5. Add the grapefruit and herbal infusion to the glass, and enjoy.

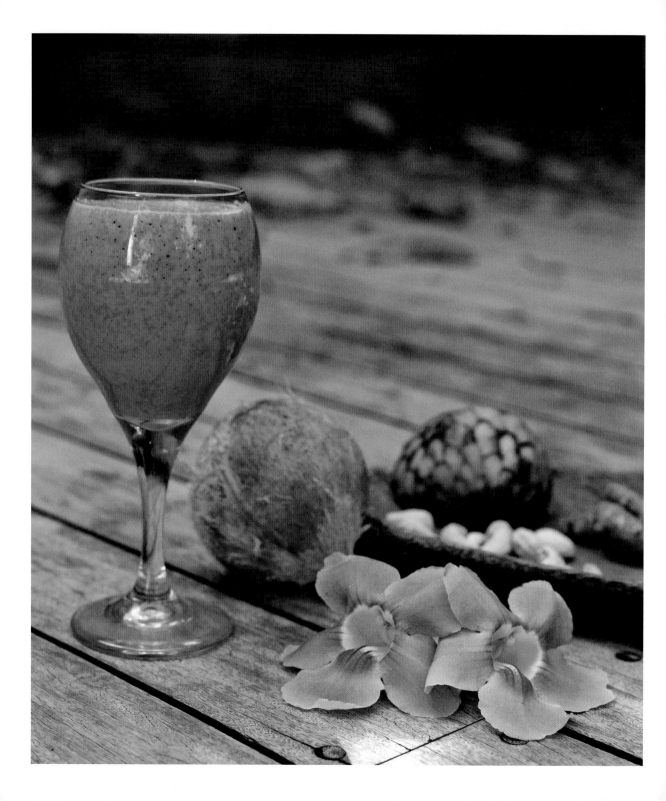

NUMBER TWO TONIC

The glory of cleaning out the intestines is unparalleled. This mix will scrape out accumulated gunk in your digestive tract and help you flush out stagnation.

Makes 1 serving

2 cups boiling water
1 teaspoon psyllium husk powder
2 teaspoons senna leaf
1 tablespoon tamarind paste
Warm water, as needed
1 cup kale
Ice
Honey or stevia to taste

Note: Senna leaves are commonly used in Central America to relieve constipation and bowel disorders. The tea cleanses the gut, relieves gas and clears stagnation from the intestines.

1. Add the boiling water to the psyllium husk and senna, and allow it to sit for about 15 minutes. Filter out the herbs and wait for the liquid to cool down.

2. In a separate container, combine the tamarind and just enough warm water to loosen it and thin the paste. Add warm water slowly to make it less pasty.

3. Once it has cooled down, add the herbal infusion into a blender, and add the kale and the tamarind preparation.

4. Add ice, and blend. Add honey to taste.

5. You'll be ready to go to the bathroom very soon!

STOMACH & INTESTINE TONER

The stomach has a slimy lining that protects us from its acids and assists us with absorption of minerals. The more this lining is damaged, the harder it is to absorb the essential nutrients that we need to thrive. Acid reflux and ulcers are examples of a disturbed digestive system due to a damaged lining. The following formula helps reset your stomach's pH and reduce inflammation in the gut.

Makes 1 serving

1 tablespoon slippery elm powder
1 tablespoon marshmallow root powder
1 tablespoon alfalfa leaf
1 tablespoon lemongrass leaf
Boiling water, as needed
1 teaspoon chia seeds
1 teaspoon lemon juice

1. In a large jar, combine the slippery elm, marshmallow root, alfalfa, and lemongrass.

2. Pour boiling water over the herbs, and allow the mixture to sit for about 45 minutes, shaking well every 10 minutes or so to activate the herbs. Use potholders to protect your hands while shaking.

3. Once the mixture has cooled to warm, add the chia seeds and lemon juice. Shake well.

4. Drink lukewarm.

MINERALIZING MOTHER TONIC

This tonic is a quick fix for stomach, liver, and kidney harmony. It is a multi-organ master mineralizing tonic. The roots and leaves it includes are known to contain some of the best sources of iron, potassium, and folic acid. Using it daily will relieve liver and gall bladder congestion, boost gut flora, and essentially provide a daily herbal vitamin.

Makes 1 "mother tonic"

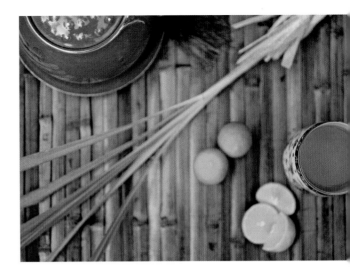

3 parts dried burdock
2 parts dried Oregon grape root
2 parts dried dandelion root
2 parts dried marshmallow root
1 parts alfalfa leaf
100 proof vodka or rum

1. Place the herbs in a wide-mouth jar, to fill about one-third of the jar.

2. Cover the herbs in vodka and allow them to soak in the liquid slowly.

3. Press the herbs down with your hand or a tool. A general rule of thumb is that if you have about 1–2 inches of liquid covering the herbs, then you have a great ratio! If the herbs still look dry, add a little more liquid.

4. To prevent rust, cover the jar with a fine cloth or plastic wrap, and place the lid on top.

5. Place in a cool, dry place, and allow 3–4 weeks for the herbs to macerate in the liquid. Shake the jar every other day.

6. Strain the liquid into a clean jar, and press the herbs in a fine-mesh cloth. Keep pressing until the herbs are basically dried out.

7. Store the tonic in a cool place, and prevent exposure to light.

Recommended dosage: 1–2 teaspoons, 2–3 times per day, or as needed.

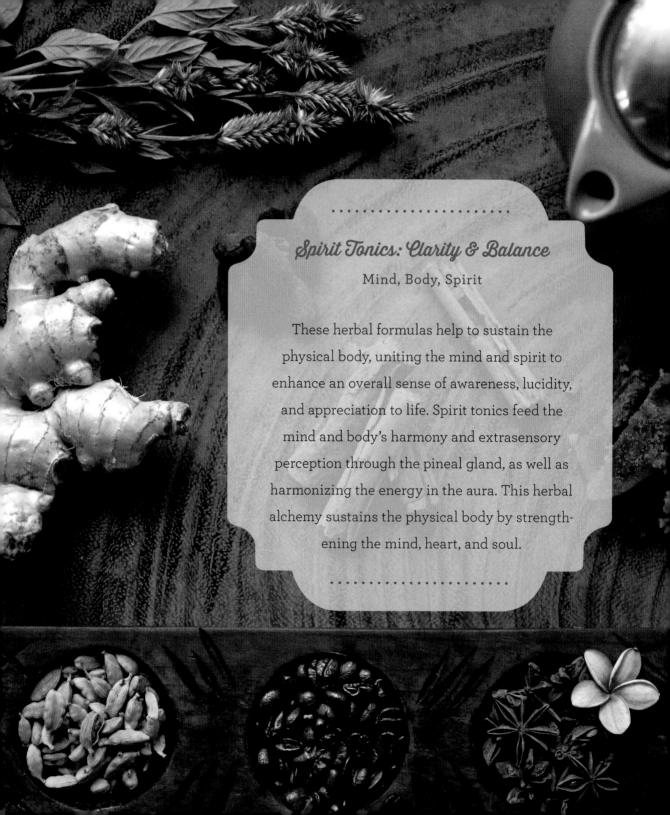

Spirit Tonics: Clarity & Balance

Mind, Body, Spirit

These herbal formulas help to sustain the physical body, uniting the mind and spirit to enhance an overall sense of awareness, lucidity, and appreciation to life. Spirit tonics feed the mind and body's harmony and extrasensory perception through the pineal gland, as well as harmonizing the energy in the aura. This herbal alchemy sustains the physical body by strengthening the mind, heart, and soul.

MEDITATION

Before entering into your meditation practice, it's lovely to soften the mind and body with a cup of relaxing tea. These herbs have been used traditionally to invoke a calming aura and bring in a feel-good atmosphere. Both have been revered as tonics for the brain and mind.

Makes 1 pot of tea

> 1 tablespoon tulsi
> 1 tablespoon skullcap
> 1 tablespoon lemon balm
> 12–14 ounces boiling water

1. Add the herbs to a teapot or tea bag, pour boiling water over them, and steep for about 10–15 minutes. Enjoy!

Alpha and Gamma Rays

Meditation and dreaming are a lot alike. They both generate alpha and gamma waves in the brain. When we activate these waves through different relaxation practices, we automatically are using a higher percentage of our brain's ability. The more we experience the presence of gamma and alpha waves throughout our day, the more we naturally live a healthier and longer life. Basically, the more relaxed we are, the happier we are.

QI RENEWAL

Qi *means "energy." In its original context,* qi *isn't simply energy; it also resembles the fine interconnected network of subtle energy that pulses through our entire body, mind, and spirit into an awake being. This formula balances the adrenals, kicks out fatigue, increases overall mind and body energy, and uplifts the spirit.*

Makes 1 pot of tea

¼ cup hemp seeds
1¾ cup warm water, divided use
1 teaspoon ashwagandha powder
1 teaspoon astragalus powder
1 teaspoon maca powder
Stevia leaf or your choice of sweetener

1. In a blender, combine the hemp seeds and ¾ cup of the water. Blend well until creamy. You can choose to either strain it or leave it whole. If you'd like the drink to be a bit less thick, strain using a fine-mesh cloth.

2. In the remaining 1 cup of warm water, add the ashwagandha, astragalus, and maca, and mix well.

3. Add the freshly made hemp milk and your choice of sweetener.

THIRD EYE TONIC

Kava and blue lotus were revered in Ancient Egypt as the herbs that invoke the gods. They have been applied in a multitude of ways, from tea to ferments to perfumes. Both have a strong and soothing chemistry, and they are known for their ability to relax the body and open the mind. This is a great tea to have before bed or to simply relax at home.

Makes 1 pot of tea

> 12–14 ounces of boiling water
> 1 teaspoon kava kava powder
> 3 tablespoons blue lotus flowers
> 3 drops chamomile essential oil

1. In a big pot, bring the water to a boil. Simmer the kava kava for about 30–45 minutes, until one-third of the water is evaporated.

2. Turn off the heat, and place a handful of blue lotus flowers in the pot. Allow them to steep about 5 minutes. Flowers are more sensitive than roots, so be sure to not cook the flowers down, because you'll lose some of their healing properties.

3. Filter out the herbs, and add the chamomile essential oil.

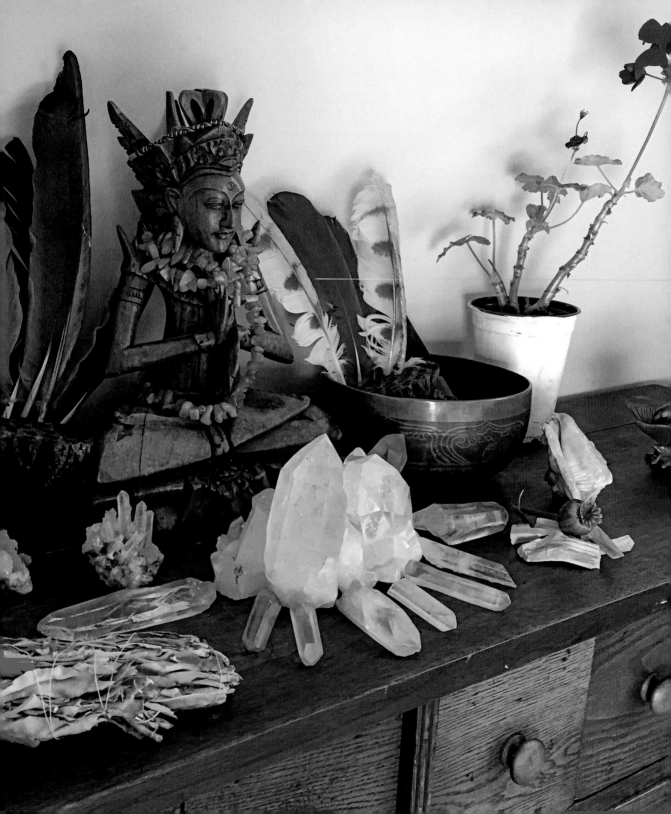

INSOMNIA'S ANTIDOTE ELIXIR

*This is a great tonic to have on hand
as an extract for treating insomnia. It
is strong and effective because it will
provide a remedy the moment you are
experiencing the insomnia. It also works
well as a tea, although it does take
time to make.* I recommend having this
extract handy whether you experience
insomnia often or not.*

*Makes 1 elixir, depending upon
amounts used.*

    3 parts dried skullcap
    3 parts dried passionflower
    2 parts dried kava kava
    1 part dried lemon balm
    100 proof vodka or rum

1. Place the herbs in a wide-mouth jar, to fill about one-third of the jar.

2. Cover the herbs in vodka, and allow them to soak in the liquid slowly.

3. Press the herbs down with your hand or a tool. A general rule of thumb is that if you have about 1–2 inches of liquid over the herbs, then you have a great ratio! If the herbs still look dry, add a little more liquid.

4. To prevent rust, cover the jar with a fine cloth or plastic wrap, and place the lid on top.

5. Place in a cool, dry place, and allow 3–4 weeks for the herbs to macerate in the liquid. Shake the jar every other day.

6. Strain the liquid into a clean jar, and press the herbs in a fine-mesh cloth. Keep pressing until the herbs are basically dried out.

7. Store the tonic in a cool place, and prevent exposure to light.

Recommended dosage: For insomnia, 1–2 tablespoons. For chronic conditions, increase the dosage as needed.

---

* The same proportions of herbs can be applied if you'd
like to make a tea instead of an elixir. Simply simmer 2
tablespoons of the herb mixture in 2 cups of water for
20 minutes. Strain, add your sweetener of choice, and enjoy.

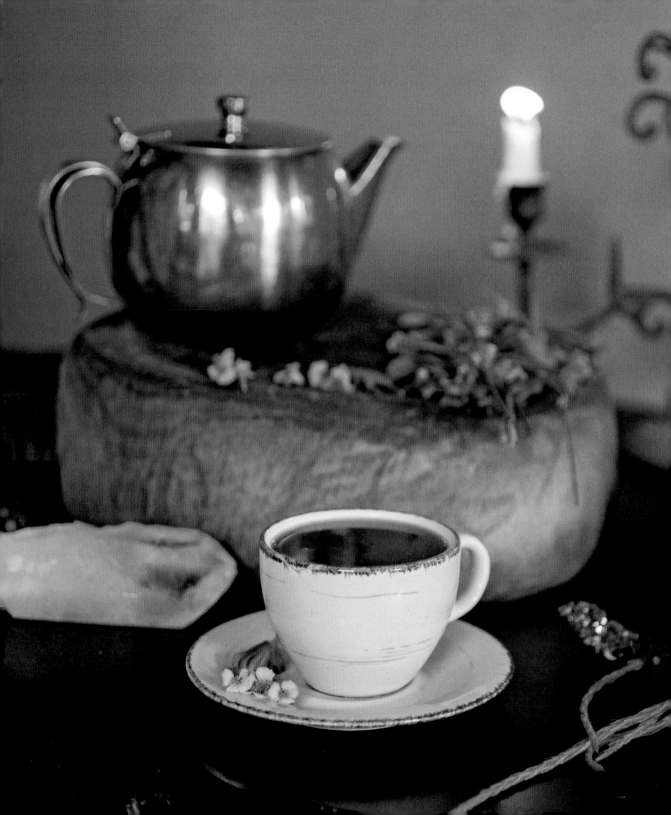

LUCID DREAMING
TEA CEREMONY*

Dream lucidity is awareness that you are dreaming. It is a mystical practice, reported since time immemorial, in which the dreamer wakes up in a dream and learns to control it by creating his or her desired outcome within the dream. These herbs have a history of decompressing the nervous system, providing a sedative quality. They provide profound relaxation. Lucid dreaming is a challenging practice, yet with persistence the results are significant.

Makes 1 pot of tea

1 teaspoon passionflower powder
1 teaspoon ashwagandha powder
1 teaspoon kava kava powder
½ teaspoon valerian powder
A pinch of mugwort leaf

16–20 ounces water
1 teaspoon blue lotus
Stevia leaf, honey, or other sweetener

Note: This recipe is an inspiration drawn from a South American recipe known to enhance *ensueño*, lucid dreaming. Many tribal peoples from the Peruvian Amazon area drink lucid dreaming tea to invoke a profound visionary state while dreaming. They believe that the alpha waves generated in dreaming, emanate from the source of where the true self lives, the third eye.

1. Add the passionflower, ashwagandha, kava kava, valerian, and mugwort to a pot with the water. Simmer for about 30 minutes.

2. Turn off the heat, and add the blue lotus.

3. Allow it to steep for 15–20 minutes without heat. Strain the herbs.

4. Add a few leaves of stevia into your brew, and mix well. Adding too much sweetness can prevent the desired effect. Keep the sugar low so the belly can relax.

---

* If you'd like to make this into an elixir, follow the same steps as the Insomnia's Antidote Elixir recipe (see page 161).

SPIRIT MOTHER TONIC

This mother tonic is an herbal mix known to enhance an overall sense of confidence, awareness, and gratefulness. This spirit blend balances the heart and mind, bringing a subtle aura of freedom and peace into the body.

Makes 1 "mother tonic"

2 parts dried tulsi
2 parts dried gotu kola
3 parts dried blue lotus
3 parts dried astragalus
100 proof vodka or rum

1. Place the herbs in a wide-mouth jar, to fill about one-third of the jar.

2. Cover the herbs in vodka and allow them to soak in the liquid slowly.

3. Press the herbs down with your hand or a tool. A general rule of thumb is that if you have about 1–2 inches of liquid going over the herbs, then you have a great ratio! If the herbs still look dry, add a little more liquid.

4. To prevent rust, cover the jar with a fine cloth or plastic wrap, and place the lid on top.

5. Place in a cool, dry place, and allow 3–4 weeks for the herbs to macerate in the liquid. Shake the jar every other day.

6. Strain the liquid into a clean jar, and press the herbs in a fine-mesh cloth. Keep pressing until the herbs are basically dried out.

7. Store the tonic in a cool place, and prevent exposure to light.

Recommended dosage: 1–2 teaspoons, 2–3 times per day, or as needed.

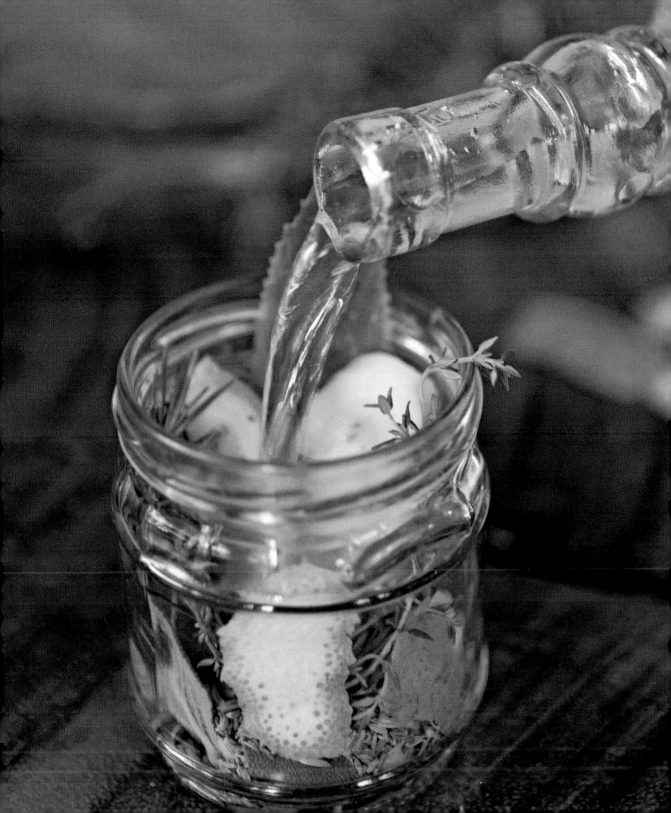

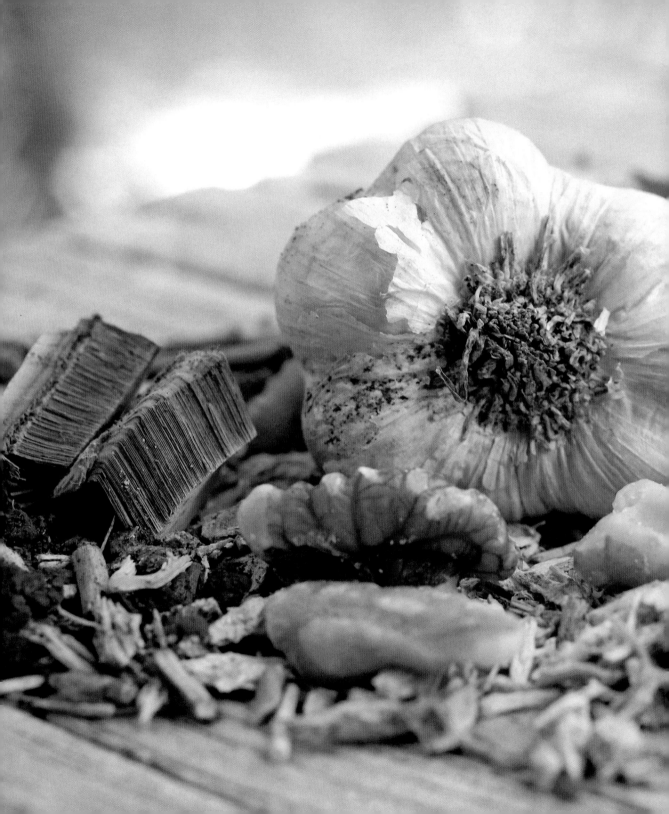

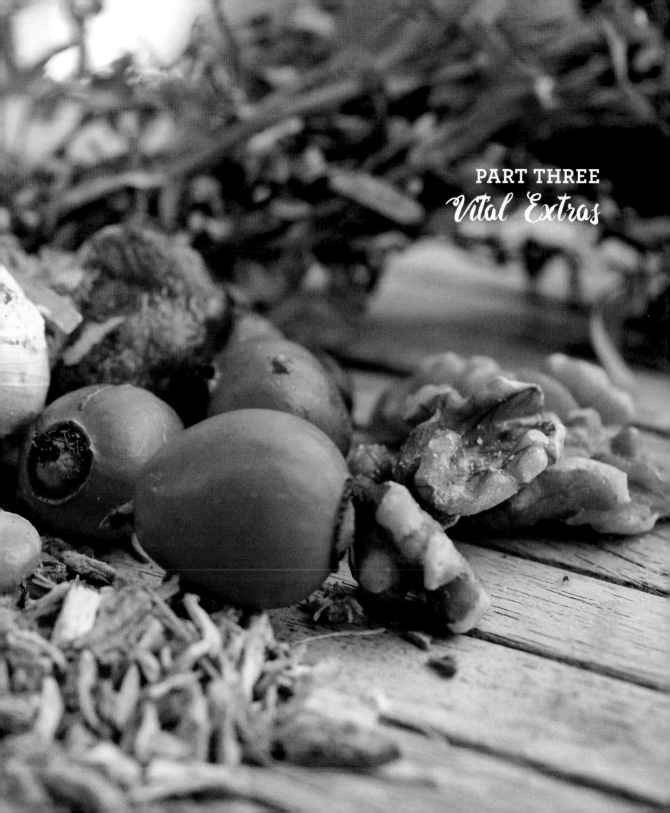

PART THREE
Vital Extras

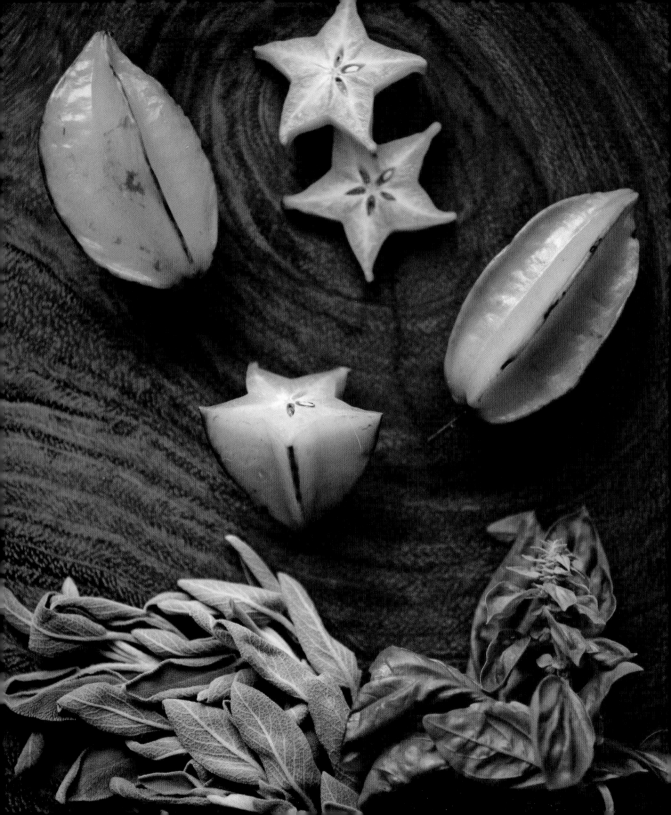

Substitutions

Nature has given us the miracle of variety and availability. You can always substitute herbs for other herbs. Some herbs may cause some side effects that you are not exactly pleased with, or you may find an inconvenience.

Be mindful about proportions, and read about the herb in this book and other suggested sources to use the right amount for you. If you are taking medications and wondering if a particular ingredient could be incompatible, the Caution section within the description should supply you with information. Always consult a health-care professional if you are dealing with a chronic disease.

Most herbs chosen for this book are absolutely safe for *most* people. I carefully chose them, keeping in mind their friendliness with different body types, as well as the ease of locating them in a store near you. Yet, still be safe and dose little by little to guide yourself in the right direction.

The chart below contain the herbs listed in the book and similar herbs you can substitute.

SUPERHERB SUBSTITUTIONS

Herb	*Substitution*
Alfalfa	Aloe, red clover, dandelion leaf
Aloe	Corn silk, slippery elm
Ashwagandha	Maca, mesquite, astragalus
Astragalus	Mesquite, fo-ti

Herb	Substitution
Black cohosh	Angelica, wild yam, vitex
Borage	Dandelion leaf, burdock
Burdock	Dandelion root, Oregon grape root
Cat's claw	Pau d'arco, jergón sacha
Chaga	Reishi, medicinal mushrooms
Chanca piedra	Moringa, graviola
Damiana	Muira puama, yohimbe
Dong quai	Wild yam
Ginkgo	Gotu kola, brahmi
Goldenseal	Ginseng (American or Chinese)
Horsetail	Comfrey
Jergón sacha	Pau d'arco
Mangosteen	Schisandra, rose hips
Marshmallow Root	Slippery elm, oats
Passionflower	Skullcap, blue lotus
Sangre de drago	Pau d'arco, jergón sacha
Saw palmetto	Papaya seeds, yohimbe
St. John's wort	Albizzia, skullcap
Suma ginseng	Siberian ginseng (eluthero)
Schisandra	Mangosteen
Senna	Cascara Sagrada, psyllium husk

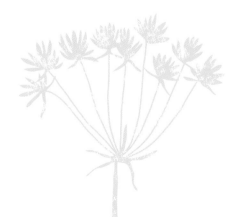

Superherb Functions

Aloe Vera *(Aloe vera)*

Parts used: Fresh leaves

Main uses and attributes:

- As a topical gel for burns, skin infections, and wounds.
- In the cosmetic world for skin and hair products, due to its alkaline nature.
- Internally normalizes digestion, alkalizing the entire gastrointestinal tract.
- Contains aloin, which acts as a natural sunscreen, blocking 30% of ultraviolet rays.
- Antiviral, particularly to combat the side effects of chronic illnesses.

Caution: Use with caution when drinking internally; overdoing it may cause diarrhea and stomach cramps.

Ashwagandha *(Withania somnifera)*

Parts used: Roots

Main uses and attributes:

- Known as India's ginseng.
- Soothes and energizes the body.
- Increases the body's overall ability to adapt to and resist stress.

- Increases memory and facilitates brain function.
- Known to restore sexual *qi* and energy, and build vital energy.
- Powerful adaptogen; reduces general debilitation, nervous tension, stress, and anxiety, infusing the body with sustainable energy.

Caution: Ashwagandha might disturb autoimmune diseases by stimulating immune activity. Patients with autoimmune diseases should be be highly cautious and use ashwagandha only under professional supervision.

Astragalus (*Astragalus membranaceus*)

Parts used: *Roots*

Main uses and attributes:

- Energizing adaptogen known to restore and regenerate immune *qi* and energy.
- Targets all major organs, particularly the spleen and lungs.
- Superior tonic herb used in the treatment of chronic illnesses.
- Stimulates the rebuilding of bone marrow reserve.
- Prevents both chronic illnesses and long-term infections.

- Promotes circulatory health and helps the body recover from radiation therapy.

Black Cohosh (*Actaea racemosa*)

Parts used: *Roots*

Main uses and attributes:

- Regulates and normalizes hormone production, acting like an estrogen "fixer."
- Known as a great nerving (nervous system relaxer) and muscle relaxant.
- Master uterus tonic; supplements the uterus with necessary minerals.
- Commonly used in formulas to balance hormone production, for general women's health, and for menopause.
- Recommended for relieving headaches and muscle spasms.

Caution: Do not use black cohosh during pregnancy, except in preparation for childbirth. Use only under professional supervision.

Borage (*Borago officinalis*)

Parts used: *Flowers, leaves, and seeds*

Main uses and attributes:

- Known to relieve anxiety and stress.
- Helps lift the spirits and relieve depression.
- As an oil, can be a great source of omega-3s and essential fatty acids.

Burdock (*Arctium lappa*)

Parts used: *Primarily roots and seeds, but leaves can be used externally*

Main uses and attributes:

- Rich in vitamins and minerals, loaded with iron, magnesium, manganese, and thiamine.
- Used primarily to detox the skin (eczema, psoriasis, acne, etc.) and liver.
- Cooling and alkalizing to the blood, being an excellent blood purifier.
- Promotes healthy kidney function and expels uric acid from the body.

Calendula (*Calendula officinalis*)

Parts used: *Flowers*

Main uses and attributes:

- Known as a master skin regenerator, promoting fast cell repair and regeneration.
- Acts as an antiseptic, keeping infection from occurring after injuries.
- Often used externally for bruises, burns, sores, digestive upsets, and skin ulcers.
- Promotes gut repair by preventing ulcers, acid reflux, indigestion, and diarrhea.

Cat's Claw (*Uncaria tomentosa*)

Parts used: *Inner bark*

Main uses and attributes:

- A powerful tonic herb that intensely targets the immune system.
- Cell repair and increasing white blood cell production.
- Treats immune disorders, gastritis, ulcers, cancer, arthritis, rheumatism, rheumatic disorders, neuralgias, and chronic inflammation of all kinds.
- Cleanses the entire intestinal tract and effective in treating digestive disorders.

- Strong immune stimulant; helps prevent strokes and heart attacks, reduce blood clots, and treat diverticulitis and irritable bowel syndrome.

Caution: *Do not use before or after an organ or bone marrow transplant since it boosts immune function. May also have a mild blood-thinning effect.*

Catuaba (*Erythroxylum catuaba*)

Parts used: *Bark*

Main uses and attributes:

- A famous Amazonian aphrodisiac considered a system stimulant.
- Relieves performance anxiety and increases sexual confidence.
- Commonly used for sexual impotency, agitation, nervousness, nerve pain and weakness, poor memory or forgetfulness, and sexual weakness.
- Acts as a great antiviral and antimicrobial.

Cayenne (*Capsicum annum*)

Parts used: *Fruits*

Main uses and attributes:

- A potent cardiotonic.
- An exquisitely spicy addition to any meal; a tiny bit goes a long way in the body, acting as an antiseptic and circulatory herb.
- Stimulates the body's natural defense system and boosts the digestive system.
- One of the best heart tonics, increasing the pulse and toning the heart muscle.
- Prevents congestion and constipation.

Caution: *Beware, it's hot! More than a pinch can overwhelm the body and irritate the gut.*

Chaga (*Inonotus obliquus*)

Parts used: *Whole fungi*

Main uses:

- A significant immune boosting medicine used by ancient peoples in Asia and Europe.
- A super-oxide dismutase (SOD) powerhouse, an important enzyme that functions as a powerful antioxidant.

- SOD chemistry performs a vital antiaging function by neutralizing oxygen free radicals, preventing oxidative damage to cells and tissues.
- Studies indicate that chaga may be beneficial as an antitumoral.
- An antioxidant- and phytonutrient-rich powerhouse.

Phyllanthus Piedra
(Phyllanthus niruri)

Parts used: *Leaf and stem*

Main uses and attributes:

- A rainforest favorite known as the "stone breaker" or "shatter stone."
- Used for generations in the Amazon.
- Known to eliminate gallstones and kidney stones.
- Used for overall liver detox and blood purification.
- A gastrointestinal tonic; reduces stomach pain, expels intestinal gas, stimulates and promotes digestion, expels worms, and acts as a mild laxative.

Chamomile *(Anthemis nobilis, Matricaria recutita)*

Parts used: *Primarily flowers, but leaves are also useful*

Main uses and attributes:

- A gentle and powerful everyday flower used for digestive harmony and relaxation.
- Known to treat colic, nervous stress, infections, and stomach acidity and disorders.
- A powerful anti-inflammatory source.
- A great calming tea, known to soothe the body, mind, and spirit.

Cinnamon *(Cinnamomum zeylanicum)*

Parts used: *Bark and essential oil*

Main uses and attributes:

- A warming digestive aid with cardiotonic properties.
- A mild stimulant; can be used to increase circulation and balance digestive problems.
- Has antiviral and antiseptic activities, making it useful for fighting infections.

Comfrey (Symphytum officinale)

Parts used: *Leaves and roots*

Main uses and attributes:

- One of the best herbs for treating strains, bruises, and any injury to the bones or joints.
- Alleviates muscle and joint spasms, bringing circulation to soft tissue.
- Known to support liver detox, although when overused it can be overtaxing to metabolize.
- A masterful skin regenerator; facilitates and activates the healing of damaged tissue.
- Soothes inflammation in the tissues and eases the liver's temper.

Damiana (Turnera aphrodisiaca)

Parts used: *Leaves*

Main uses and attributes:

- A restorative herb to the reproductive system, increasing sexual vitality.
- Revitalizes exhausted nerves, exhausted reproductive system, and exhausted spirit.
- Acts as a relaxant and antidepressant.
- Boosts sexual vitality and ability, increasing a euphoric state of being.

- Helps impotence, infertility, nervous exhaustion, anxiety, performance anxiety, and other depressive factors within sexual matters.

Dandelion (Taraxacum officinale)

Parts used: *Leaves, roots, and flowers*

Main uses and attributes:

- A restorative and rejuvenating herb to the liver and gut.
- Induces the flow of bile and cleaning the liver, gall bladder, and portal vein.
- A safe diuretic, known to tone the kidneys and aid in proper water elimination.
- Leaves are high in vitamins and minerals, including calcium, magnesium, iron, and vitamins A and C.

Dong Quai (Angelica sinensis)

Part used: *Root*

Main uses and attributes:

- Known as the "the female ginseng."
- An excellent root for strengthening and balancing the uterus.
- Nourishes the blood and has a mellow cleansing and stimulating action on the liver.

- Assists the liver and endocrine system; regulates hormonal production.
- Used for menstrual irregularities; stimulates menstrual bleeding.

Caution: Not recommended during menstruation or for the duration of pregnancy. If you take dong quai over an extended period, discontinue its use one week before the onset of menses, resuming after menstruation has ceased.

Echinacea *(Echinacea angustifolia, E. purpurea, E. pallida)*

Parts used: *Roots, leaves, and flowers*

Main uses and attributes:

- A master immunestimulant; also acts as a decongestant and facilitates sinus relief.
- Increases T-cell activity, thereby boosting the body's first line of defense against colds, flus, and many other illnesses.
- Prevents and treats colds, boosting the body with antibodies.

Fennel *(Foeniculum vulgare)*

Parts used: *Primarily seeds (flowers and leaves are used as well)*

Main uses and attributes:

- An exquisite digestive aid; expels gas and alleviates other gut imbalances.
- An antacid, neutralizing excess acids in the stomach and intestines.
- Known to increase and enrich milk flow in nursing mothers.

Feverfew *(Tanacetum parthenium)*

Parts used: *Leaves and flowers*

Main uses and attributes:

- Popularly known to heal and prevent migraine headaches and common headaches; its action is similar to that of aspirin, with a stronger but slower effect.
- Assists in relieving upper body inflammation and stress-related tension.
- Inhibits the production of prostaglandins, which are implicated in inflammation, swelling, and PMS.

Fo-ti (*Polygonum multiflorum*)

Parts used: *Roots*

Main uses and attributes:

- Known as the beautifying adaptogen.
- Restores overall vitality.
- Increases healthy hair and nail growth.
- Popular longevity herb.
- Enhances sexual energy.
- Specific for cleansing the liver.
- Strengthens kidney *qi*.
- Relaxing and is useful during times of stress and anxiety, despite being a great tonic and energizer.
- Contains resveratrol and lecithin, two compounds that have a beneficial effect on cholesterol levels and enhance circulatory function.

Garlic (*Allium sativum*)

Parts used: *Bulbs*

Main uses and attributes:

- A potent internal and external antiseptic.
- Stimulates the body's immune system.
- Well known for expelling intestinal worms.

- Helps maintain healthy blood cholesterol levels and lower high blood pressure.

Ginger (*Zingiber officinale*)

Parts used: *Roots*

Main uses and attributes:

- Essential for the digestive system; a must-have harmonizer.
- Used in formulas to tie in the flavor profile and provide healing groundwork to any combination.
- Improves poor circulation in all major areas of the body.
- A good diaphoretic that opens up the pores and promotes sweat.
- Improves digestion and helps the body efficiently move out waste.

Ginkgo (*Ginkgo biloba*)

Parts used: *Leaves and fruit*

Main uses and attributes:

- Enhances memory, vitality, and circulation.
- Improves circulation and vasodilatation, making it an energizing and anti-inflammatory remedy.

- Popularly used for the cerebral region, from ear to eye to brain imbalances.
- Acts as a strong antioxidant and useful against free radicals, substances that damage cellular health and accelerate aging.
- Serves as a cardiac tonic by increasing the strength of the arterial walls.
- Promotes blood flow and oxygenation throughout the body, which makes it an essential everyday longevity tonic.

Ginseng, American (*Panax quinquefolius*)

Parts used: Roots

Main uses and attributes:

- A phenomenal immune-boosting adaptogen.
- Cools, nourishes, and soothes the system.
- A great overall balancing tonic for the entire body; targets all five major organ systems.
- Restores energy and repairs exhausted *qi* reservoirs.
- Treats general debilitation, increases mental clarity, and is an excellent source of minerals and vitamins.

Ginseng, Asian (*Panax ginseng*)

Parts used: Roots

Main uses and attributes:

- An ancient "cure-all," and long renowned as master adaptogen.
- Superior adaptogenic strength helps the body resist a wide spectrum of illnesses.
- When used over a period of time, revitalizes and restores energy and is especially good for building sexual vitality.
- A great reproductive tonic for men and women.
- Rejuvenates the entire nervous system, regenerates overtaxed nerves, and discourages mood swings and depression.

Graviola (*Annona muricata*)

Parts used: Leaf, bark, fruit, and seeds

Main uses and attributes:

- Popularly known as a nourishing and mineralizing tonic to the digestive system.
- Known to have strong anticancerous chemistry and a miraculous ability to support radiation recovery.
- Crushed seeds are used for worms and parasites.

- Heals the gut from overall bad bacteria buildup.

Gotu Kola *(Centella asiatica)*

Parts used: *Leaves*

Main uses and attributes:

- A magnificent brain herb, known to repair cerebral imbalance.
- Recommended for memory loss; increases mental activity and focus.
- Successfully used in treatment programs for epilepsy, schizophrenic behavior, and Alzheimer's disease.
- Superb in formulas for nervous stress and debility.

Hibiscus *(Hibiscus sabdariffa)*

Parts used: *Flowers and sometimes leaves*

Main uses and attributes:

- High in vitamin C and bioflavonoids.
- An exquisite astringent and diuretic source.
- Useful for treating mild colds, flus, bruising, and swelling.
- Used in fat-burner formulas to support weight loss.

Jergón Sacha *(Dracontium lorotense)*

Parts used: *Roots*

Main uses and attributes:

- Taken for viral infections, candida, and fungal infections.
- Known as an anticancer and potent antiviral fighter.
- Aids in gastrointestinal problems, hernias (as a decoction applied topically), hand tremors, and heart palpitations, while enhancing immune function.

Kava Kava *(Piper methysticum)*

Parts used: *Roots*

Main uses and attributes:

- Total body relaxant; heightens awareness and makes you feel brighter.
- Reduces tension, anxiety, and stress.
- Analgesic properties alleviate pain and assist the mind in relaxing in times of stress.
- Supports calming of long-term stress and anxiety.

Lavender (*Lavandula spp.*)

Parts used: *Flowers*

Main uses and attributes:

- A magnificent flower with strong relaxing properties.
- Acts as a mild antidepressant and offers great relief for headache sufferers.
- Combined with feverfew, helps alleviate migraines.
- One of the best herbs for alleviating tension, stress, and insomnia.
- Essential oil is an excellent antibacterial and antiviral.

Lemon Balm (*Melissa officinalis*)

Parts used: *Leaves and flowers*

Main uses and attributes:

- A gentle and calming leaf known for its antiseptic nature.
- Strong antispasmodic effect on the stomach and nervous system.
- An excellent remedy for stomach distress and general exhaustion.
- Commonly used as a mild sedative and for insomnia.

Licorice (*Glycyrrhiza glabra*)

Parts used: *Roots*

Main uses and attributes:

- An outstanding tonic for the endocrine system.
- Particularly effective for relieving adrenal exhaustion.
- Natural antidepressive and digestive regulator.
- Regarded as a remedy for the respiratory system; used as a soothing demulcent and anti-inflammatory remedy for respiratory problems.

Lycium aka Goji Berries (*Lycium chinense*)

Parts used: *Berries*

Main uses and attributes:

- Known as a longevity tonic.
- Enhances kidney function and blood mineralization.
- Assist liver detox and spleen function.
- A circulatory aid; used as a blood tonic.

Marshmallow Root
(Althaea officinalis)

Parts used: Primarily roots, but leaves and flowers are useful

Main uses and attributes:

- A soothing mucilaginous herb used to rebuild the guts mucilaginous walls.
- Eases acidity; used to prevent ulcers.
- Commonly used for sore throats, diarrhea, constipation, and bronchial inflammation.

Milk Thistle *(Silybum marianum)*

Parts used: Seeds; leaves can be eaten (watch out for the thorns!)

Main uses and attributes:

- A powerful antioxidant with potent detoxification properties.
- Expels toxic buildup in the body, releasing stagnation from the liver and blood.
- Helps fight the damaging effects of free radicals, relinquishing the effects of many age-related diseases.
- Rebuilds liver cells that have been damaged by illness, rich food, hepatitis, or alcohol consumption.
- Protects the liver against damaging chemicals.

- Helpful for the gallbladder and the kidneys.

Moringa *(Moringa oleifera)*

Parts used: Commonly seed and leaf

Main uses and attributes:

- Excellent source of nutrition and natural energy booster.
- Leaf helps lower blood pressure.
- Nature's multivitamin; provides seven times the vitamin C of oranges, four times the calcium of milk, four times the vitamin A of carrots, three times the potassium of bananas, and two times the protein of yogurt.
- Miracle tree known for its strengthening and energizing nature.

Muira Puama *(Ptychopetalum olacoides, Liriosma ovata)*

Parts used: Bark

Main uses and attributes:

- A well-loved aphrodisiac throughout South America.
- Supports those suffering from impotence and depressed sexual activity.
- A highly regarded sexual stimulant also known to increase euphoria and joy.

- Mode of action is unknown at this time, but seems to have no side effects.
- Used to treat dysentery, diarrhea, and other diseases for which a strong astringent is indicated.

Nettle *(Urtica dioica)*

Parts used: Leaves, seeds, roots, and young tops

Main uses and attributes:

- A superior tonic that is a true mineral factory—rich in iron, calcium, potassium, silicon, magnesium, manganese, zinc, and chromium.
- Strengthens and tones the entire system; known to restore vital energy and mineralize the blood.
- Boosts kidney function, uplifting the spirit.
- Promotes liver cleansing.
- Assists in hypoallergic imbalances, preventing hay fever.

Oats *(Avena sativa)*

Parts used: Green milky tops, seeds, and stalks

Main uses and attributes:

- An exquisite nerve tonic with a cardiotonic supportive nature.
- A great food source for those who are overworked, stressed, or anxious.
- Provides energy by increasing overall health and vitality.
- Frequently used for nervous system disorders, depression, anxiety, and low vitality.
- Natural mucilaginous properties make it particularly helpful to the gut lining and the myelin sheath, which covers and protects nerve fibers.
- One of the best sources of magnesium within the herbal world.

Oregon Grape
(Mahonia aquifolium)

Parts used: Roots

Main uses and attributes:

- Roots contain berberine, a compound known for its anti-inflammatory and antiseptic abilities.
- A strong antiviral.

- An excellent source for fighting infection and topical cleansing, making it especially useful for treating skin conditions such as acne, eczema, and psoriasis.
- A fantastic blood builder; assists the liver and gall bladder in cleansing and removing heavy metals.

Passionflower
(Passiflora incarnata)

Part used: Leaves and flowers

Main uses and attributes:

- A calming and relaxing herb known to decompress the nervous system.
- Known to treat epilepsy, anxiety, insomnia, and panic attacks.
- Effective as a mild pain reliever.
- Strong antispasmodic actions, which make it useful for headaches, cramps, and muscle spasms.
- Well known for its sleep-inducing properties.
- One of the best herbs for stress, anxiety, and depression.

Peppermint *(Mentha piperita)*

Parts used: Leaves and flowers

Main uses and attributes:

- A cooling agent with powerful antimicrobial properties.
- Commonly used as a digestive aid; eases and cools the digestive process and soothes the intestines.

Rose Hips *(Rosa canina and Other Species)*

Parts used: Primarily seeds, but also leaves and flowers

Main uses and attributes:

- Contain more vitamin C than almost any other herb.
- A noted antioxidant with disease-fighting abilities.
- Used in cosmetics for its potent hair and skin regenerative qualities.

Rosemary *(Rosmarinus officinalis)*

Parts used: Leaves

Main uses and attributes:

- Popularly used as a memory aid.
- Has a tonic effect on the nervous system.

- Strengthens the heart and reduces high blood pressure.
- Acts as a strong antimicrobial, and great for fighting colds and flus.

Sangre de Drago *(Croton lechleri)*

Parts used: Tree resin and bark

Main uses and attributes:

- A liquid resin painted on wounds to staunch bleeding.
- Accelerates healing.
- Acts as a great internal and external bandage, preventing bleeding and hemorrhages; commonly used externally by indigenous tribes and local people in Peru for wounds, fractures, and hemorrhoids, and used internally for intestinal and stomach ulcers.
- Other indigenous peoples use it as an anticancer and digestive healer.

St. John's Wort *(Hypericum perforatum)*

Parts used: Leaves and flowers

Main uses and attributes:

- Popularly used to treat depression and anxiety.
- A classic healer to assist in repairing nerve damage, depression, personality disorders, and other psychological imbalances.
- Assists in treatment of damage to the nerve endings such as in burns, neuralgia, wounds, and trauma to the skin.
- Relieves the symptoms of stress, anxiety, depression, and chronic fatigue; increasing a sense of euphoria and happiness.

Caution: Please see a professional if you are taking antidepressants or nerve-related pharmaceuticals. It may cause misinteractions. Please be careful and dose yourself wisely.

Saw Palmetto *(Serenoa repens)*

Parts used: Berries

Main uses and attributes:

- One of the best remedies for inflammation of the prostate gland.
- Strengthening to those individuals who are continually nervous and stressed and who lack energy and vitality.
- Known for its great ability to assist the prostate and nourish the kidneys and bladder with essential minerals and vitamins.

Schisandra (Schisandra chinensis)

Part used: Berries

Main uses and attributes:

- An adaptogenic master herb, known to boost the body with energy and relieve stress and disease.
- Increases endurance and stamina, builds the immune system, supports the heart, and protects the liver, while harmonizing the digestive system.
- Often used for the lungs and respiratory illnesses.
- Contains the five flavors, known to target the five main organs.
- Known to assist in regulating and balancing major hormonal systems.

Senna (Cassia angustifolia)

Parts used: Leaves and pods

Main uses and attributes:

- A common and very popular laxative.
- Used in Ayurvedic medicine for liver, skin, and respiratory problems.
- Clears the intestines of excess accumulation and cleanses the entire digestive tract.

Caution: Senna should not be used over long periods of time, as it will weaken the bowels and create a dependency, but it is very useful for acute cases of constipation.

Skullcap (Scutellaria lateriflora)

Parts used: Leaves

Main uses and attributes:

- A great and tasty relaxing pain reliever.
- A versatile nervine indicated for nervous system disorders, especially headaches, nerve tremors, stress, insomnia, and nervous exhaustion.
- Commonly used as an analgesic, often used for PMS and lower belly pain.

Slippery Elm (Ulmus fulva, U. rubra)

Parts used: Inner bark

Main uses and attributes:

- A soothing mucilaginous herb known to calm gut-related inflammation.
- Can be used internally or externally.
- Particularly valuable for burns, sore throats, and digestive problems, including diarrhea and constipation.
- A highly nourishing food that is a great mineralizer and gut flora replenisher.

Stevia *(Stevia rebaudiana)*

Parts used: *Leaves*

Main uses and attributes:

- Sweeter than sugar but much better for you; has no calories and doesn't promote tooth decay.
- Used for pancreatic imbalances and high blood sugar levels.
- A type of sugar that diabetics can tolerate.
- Stevia has been used to help treat diabetes and other blood sugar–related imbalances.

Turmeric *(Curcuma longa)*

Parts used: *Roots*

Main uses and attributes:

- Clinically proven to be a remarkable anti-inflammatory, antioxidant, and vitamin C source.
- Popularly used as a skin tonic and an agent to draw out inflammation out of soft tissue, muscles, and joints.
- Used as an anticancer, cholagogueue, and depurative (herbs help cleanse waste products and toxins from our body, and are a staple of traditional herbal medicine).

- Contains potent diuretic and kidney-cleansing properties, assisting the liver and gall bladder in detoxing, while relieving the gut and being a great wound healer.

Valerian *(Valeriana officinalis)*

Parts used: *Roots*

Main uses and attributes:

- A highly regarded sedative.
- A great stress reliever, preventing insomnia and nervous system disorders.
- Has powerful tonic effects on the heart and is often recommended with circulatory herbs to enhance its strength.

Wild Yam *(Dioscorea villosa)*

Parts used: *Rhizomes and roots*

Main uses and attributes:

- Serves as a hormone precursor, aiding the proper function of the reproductive system of both sexes.
- Supports menstrual harmony and increases fertility.
- Oddly, sometimes listed as a natural birth control agent, though it is more often used to promote fertility.

- Bitter compounds tone the liver and enhance the blood with nourishment.
- Wild yam is excellent for soothing muscle cramps, colic, and uterine pain.

Witch Hazel
(Hamamelis virginiana)

Parts used: Bark

Main uses and attributes:

- An astringent external liniment and astringent, disinfectant wash.
- A potent pain reliever with antioxidant properties.
- Thought to act on the venous system to stop bleeding and inflammation.

Yohimbe *(Pausinystalia yohimbe, Corynanthe yohimbe)*

Parts used: Shavings of the inner bark

Main uses and attributes:

- A very potent aphrodisiac and stimulant.
- Stimulates blood flow to the reproductive organs, particularly to the penis.
- Yohimbine hydrochloride, a product sold by pharmaceutical companies, is a prescription drug used for treating erectile dysfunction. It can also be used—with caution—to increase libido.

Caution: Use wisely. It can be damaging if overdone or taken in large doses. Speak with your health provider.

Where Do I Find These Ingredients?

Sourcing ingredients is an ongoing adventure. I'm the kind of person who likes to constantly search for new regions and new farmers producing one-of-a-kind herbs and foods. Sometimes I find myself in a pinch when supply is low because harvest is done for the year, or I am traveling and it's not easy to bring ingredients with me, or the local market doesn't carry what I'm looking for. Try to remember these basic keys when buying your superfoods.

FRESH IS ALWAYS BEST.

No matter what, fresh is always best. Don't worry about not being able to find an ingredient or not being able to afford it. There are always alternatives. The fresher and most local ingredient to you will be 10 times healthier for you than sourcing from the other side of the world. Of course, there are rare plant species in the rainforest that are one of a kind, and it is a true delight and miracle that we are able to purchase them and store them in our kitchen cabinet. Indulge in these aspects of modern living, but also honor the seasons and local availability as much as possible. Sometimes you'd be amazed what you can find around you!

GO TO YOUR LOCAL FARMERS MARKET.

You may find a farmer at your market that is growing the herb you are looking for. Most farmers markets around the world have common herbs and superfoods, such as lavender, mint, sage, rosemary, oregano, thyme, and so on. These are very easy to find; always choose fresh versus dry for the common ones. Same goes for mushrooms; you can usually find oysters, turkey tail, maitake, shiitake, and agarics (white button), and, depending on location, reishi, chaga, lions mane, and so on. Always use fresh for the ones you are able to find. Ask farmers if they happen to have other varieties of herbs available within their farm. Many times they do, and they probably would love to supply you with what you are requesting, or maybe even grow it especially for you.

ALWAYS GO ORGANIC AND SUSTAINABLE.

Organic these days is perhaps not as organic as we wish it would be. Some farmers are not organically certified yet have the best and most nourishing availability. Meet your farmer, or ask your source. Plenty of people are on the quest for purity. Ask about their sourcing or form of growing medicines. In Latin America, for example, particularly in the area of herbs, most of the time the herbs are wildcrafted. Families survive on living close to the rainforest, harvesting what is around, and bringing it to the market.

WILDCRAFT YOUR MEDICINE!

Wildcrafting is a way of life. No matter where you live or what you do, there is always a nearby place you can go to pick your own herbs. Try finding a beautiful hike that is not close to any highway or waste area, and pick the weeds and herbs you may find along the way. There is no doubt that you'll find medicinal herbs. There are many foraging guides; look for one that targets your area and learn about the herbs and weeds that grow around you. You'll become a wildcrafting master in no time!

EXPLORE ONLINE MARKETPLACES

There are fantastic online sources that have a large collection of truly organic, fair trade, and biodynamic superherbs and herbal products. I recommend researching your favorite places, initiating a conversation about where and how they make their products, and choosing for yourself. In the Resources section you can find my favorite places to find raw materials and ready-made products.

Resources

KITCHEN TOOLS

Amazon
www.amazon.com
Any tool or shelf-stable ingredient you can't find locally, such as nut milk bags, fine-mesh cloths, mixing spoons, blender parts replacements, and so on.

Breville
www.brevilleusa.com
High-quality kitchen equipment.

Champion Juicer
www.championjuicer.com
The best masticating juicer available.

Norwalk Juicer
www.norwalkjuicers.com
The best home-scale cold-pressing machine.

Specialty Bottle
www.specialtybottle.com
Containers, jars, and herbal extract storage bottles.

Vitamix
www.vitamix.com
Blending master machines.

HERBS AND TONICS

Healing Spirits Herb Farm and Education Center
www.healingspiritsherbfarm.com
One of the best sources in the Northeast of ethically wild-crafted and organically grown herbs.

Herbs Frontier Natural Products Co-op
www.frontiercoop.com
A giant supplier of herbs and natural products.

Horizon Herbs
www.strictlymedicinalseeds.com
The best medicinal herbs seed collection.

Monterey Spice Co.
www.herbco.com
Herbal company offering lots of bulk herbs.

Mountain Rose Herbs
www.mountainroseherbs.com
An herbal company offering organic, vegan, kosher, and fair-trade herbs, superfoods, and other herbal products.

StarWest Botanicals (formerly Trinity Herbs)
www.starwest-botanicals.com
Bulk herb.

TropiLab
www.tropilab.com
Exporter and wholesaler of medicinal plants, herbs, tropical seeds, and cut flowers from the Amazon in Suriname.

Wild Weeds
www.wildweeds.com
Organically grown herbs and cosmetic ingredients.

Zack Woods Herb Farm
www.zackwoodsherbs.com
Owned and operated by Rosemary Gladstar's daughter Melanie and her husband, Jeff, Zach Woods supplies some of the finest organic dried herbs available.

HERBAL PRODUCTS

Anima Mundi Herbals
www.animamundiherbals.com
A rainforest apothecary made by Adriana Ayales, featuring one-of-a-kind high-potency tonics, elixirs, and superfood formulas.

Avena Botanicals
www.avenabotanicals.com
A range of organic herbal products.

Blue Bonnet Nutrition
www.bluebonnetnutrition.com
For overall supplements, supplement oils, and herbal capsules.

Floracopeia
www.floracopeia.com
An extraordinary collection of essential oils, infusers, and flowers essences.

Herbalist and Alchemist
www.herbalist-alchemist.com
A full line of Western and Chinese herbs and formulations.

Herb Pharm
www.herb-pharm.com
A comprehensive line of high-quality herbal extracts.

Host Defense
www.hostdefense.com
A company founded by Paul Stamets that offers mushroom supplements.

Sambazon
www.sambazon.com
A source for fresh frozen rainforest fruits: acai, acerola, camu camu, capuaca.

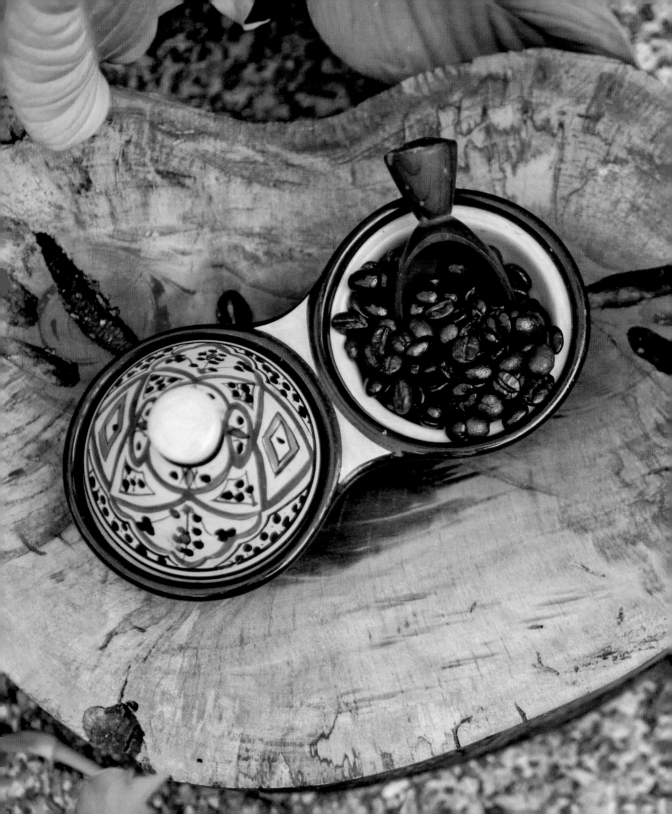

References

Beryl, Paul. *A Compendium of Herbal Magick*. Custer, WA: Phoenix Publishing, 1998.

Cech, Richo. *Making Plant Medicine*. 3rd ed. Williams, OR: Horizon Herbs, 2014.

Cousens, Gabriel. *Spiritual Nutrition*. Berkeley, CA: North Atlantic Books, 1987, 2005.

———. *There Is a Cure for Diabetes*. Berkeley, CA: North Atlantic Books, 2008.

Gladstar, Rosemary. *Herbal Recipes for Vibrant Health*. North Adams, MA: Storey Publishing, 2010.

———. *Medicinal Herbs*. North Adam, MA: Storey Publishing, 2012.

Green, James. *The Herbal Medicine-Maker's Handbook: A Home Manual*. Berkeley, CA: Crossing Press, 2011.

Grieve, Margaret. *A Modern Herbal, Volume I & II*. New York: Dover Publications, 1971.

Gurudas. *Gem Elixirs and Vibrational Healing Volume I & II*. 1st ed. San Rafael, CA: Cassandra Press, 1986.

———. *Spiritual Properties of Herbs*. San Rafael, CA: Cassandra Press, 1988.

Hoffman, David. *Medical Herbalism*. Rochester, VT: Healing Arts Press, 2003.

Lad, Vasant. *Ayurveda: The Science of Self-Healing.* Twin Lakes, WI: Lotus Press, 1984.

Lad, Vasant, and David Frawley. *Yoga of Herbs.* Santa Fe: Lotus Press, 1986.

Taylor, Leslie. *The Healing Power of Rainforest Herbs.* Garden City Park, NY: Square One Publishers, 2005.

Tierra, Michael. *The Way of Herbs.* New York: Washington Square Press, 1983.

Wigmore, Ann. *The Hippocrates Diet and Health Program.* New York: Avery Publishing, 1983.

Winston, David. *Adaptogens: Herbs for Strength, Stamina, and Stress Relief.* Rochester, VT: Healing Arts Press, 2010.

Wolfe, David. *Eating for Beauty.* Berkeley, CA: North Atlantic Books, 2007.

———. *Superfoods: The Food and Medicine of the Future.* Berkeley, CA: North Atlantic Books, 2009.

Wood, Mathew. *The Book of Herbal Wisdom: Using Plants as Medicines.* Berkeley, CA: North Atlantic Books, 1997.

INTERNET RESOURCES

American Indian Ethnobotany Database

http://herb.umd.umich.edu

A database of Native American foods, drugs, dyes, and fibers derived from plants.

HerbMed Database

www.herbmed.org

An online herbal database that provides links to the scientific data underlying the use of herbs for health. It is an evidence-based information resource for professionals, researchers, and the general public.

Leslie Taylor
Raintree Database
www.rain-tree.com/plist.htm#.Vj5WMc4y-qA
A doctor and rainforest herbalist mastermind. A complete and fully studied
database of the most popular rainforest herbs.

PubMed
www.ncbi.nlm.nih.gov/pubmed
National Library of Medicine's search interface to access the 10 million citations in
Medline, Pre-Medline, and other related databases.

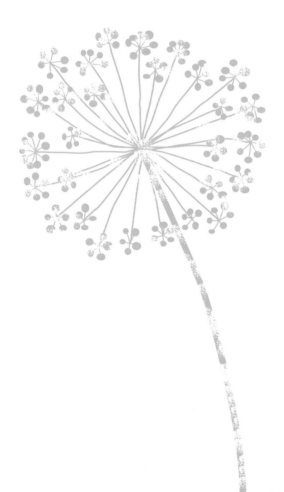

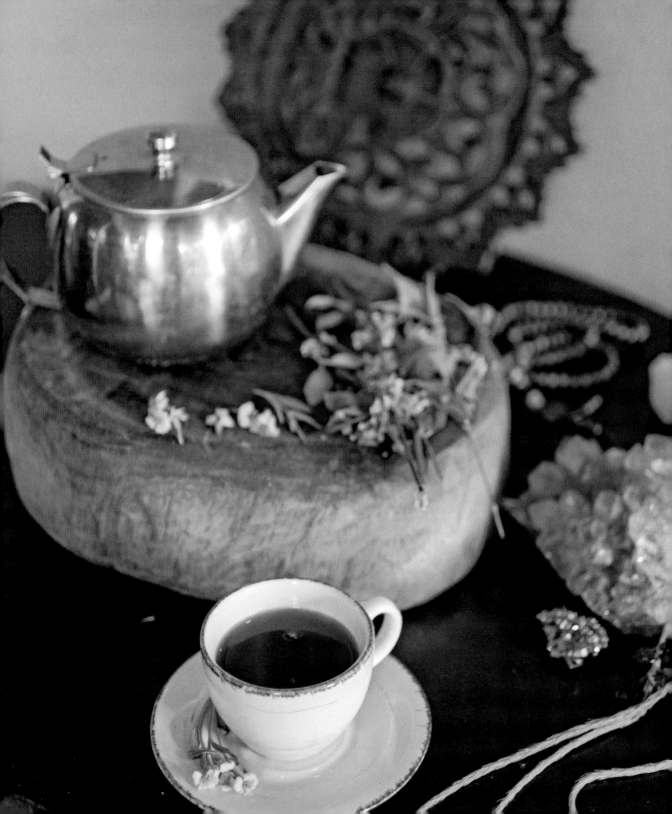

Acknowledgments

I'm so incredibly fortunate to have such fun, creative, and powerful people in the community.

I'm beyond grateful to Jennifer Harter for making the book come alive with her wonderful photography. The love and devotion put into art, food, and placement shines through, and I cherish the time spent creating with her.

My wonderful and supporting family has instilled in me an authentic and creative approach to living. It's because of them that I've been fearlessly following my dream, and simply going for this path. Especially my dear loving mother, who has always believed in my wild dreams since I was young.

Thank you to my beloved partner, who supports me through long hours of writing, blogging, and medicine making/tasting/creating. From mixing giant barrels of tonics to finding the perfect wood surface to make medicine on, you are the best.

Thank you to the Sterling Publishing team for making such an amazing project come alive. An incredible way of life is now made available to everyone, thanks to you. This is an incredible first of many pieces of written art to come.

About the Author

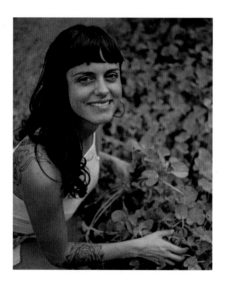

Adriana Ayales is a Costa Rican native with the passion to restore the secrets of ancient botany. From a young age she has dedicated herself to the study of plants and healing. Her background integrates rainforest tribal-style botany, as well as classic European alchemy. Her expertise is in bridging the healing cosmologies between indigenous medicine and Western practices. Her formulas infuse biodynamic and organically sourced herbs from the most pristine places on the planet. She lives in New York City.

Index

Page numbers in *italics* indicate illustrations.

(continued on the
following page)

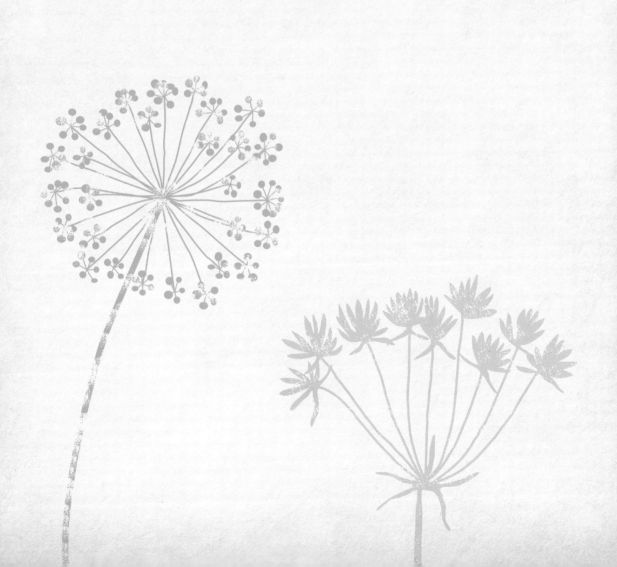